career, kids and breast cancer

A breast cancer diary

Joanna Anthony

Pen Press Publishers Ltd

First published in Great Britain
Imprint: Indepenpress

Pen Press Publishers Ltd
39-41 North Road
London N7 9DP

ISBN 1 905203-37-3
Second edition

A catalogue record for this book is available
from the British Library

Printed and bound in Great Britain

Cover design by Colin Anthony
Photography by Gary Sandy

Dedicated to

Colin
*Thank you for your incredible strength
and support*

Grace and Eliot
Love the life you live

Contents

Heartfelt thanks to…
Who does what in the cancer care world

Foreword

This is my account of my brush with breast cancer, relating my experience of the treatment that you undergo following a diagnosis, detailing the questions – and some answers – that you ask yourself.

It is important to understand that my experience is unique, just as yours is – each person facing cancer treatment is treated differently and reacts differently to the different treatments. The bits I found hardest going may be easy for some people; some of my treatments won't be relevant to your individual case, and equally I won't be offered some of the treatments that you may be offered.

I have written this book to help people facing treatment for cancer, and to help their partners and loved ones. I believe it will help all people involved to understand both the functional and emotional aspects to cancer. If you're just looking for factual information, read the newspaper articles; if you're seeking a more emotional viewpoint, read the diary. If you want as much information as possible, just read both.

The diary sets out some of the questions that I raised, to help you identify what questions you want to ask. So often I was asked if I had any questions – certainly I sought loads of answers, but I didn't know what questions I needed to ask to get to the answer.

The newspaper & magazine articles illustrate the views of the day across a wide range of issues, and demonstrate the huge leaps that are being made in cancer treatment just over the course of one year. The information will date, but the referenced companies and websites will remain up to the minute, so use the reference list to keep up to speed with the developments in breast cancer treatment.

I have drawn conclusions about my personal views on the different issues, as well as putting forward advice on how I coped with the different treatments, and the varied reactions to treatment.

I really hope this helps you.

PART I

Chapter One
The Longest Day

Friday 18th February, 3pm

'We have found a lump, and think it is highly suspicious,' the doctor said, looking up from my newly created case notes which comprised one piece of paper in a yellow folder, marked up with my name and a freshly-issued hospital number.

I held my breath, waiting for him to continue. What on earth did he mean, 'highly suspicious'? I kept looking at him, my vision getting blurred as I continued to hold my breath, but my senses seemed to sharpen as my brain registered the scene... the middle-aged consultant surgeon on the other side of the large, plain, utilitarian wooden desk, in front of a wide and rather dirty window that looked out onto the irregular shapes of other hospital buildings; the flat, greyness of the February sky, and of the three nurses on the other side of the large, clinical consulting room who also seemed to be holding their breath, waiting for me to... to what? All eyes were on me.

'Are you alright?' the consultant asked gently, leaning forward and looking at me closely.

I breathed. 'I don't know. Did you just tell me that I had a malignant tumour?' my voice echoed in my head, seeming to come from a long way off.

He nodded.

'Then I'm not alright, am I?' My voice sounded sarcastic and hard this time. But it wasn't me controlling its pitch and tone. The doctor sat back, as though I'd gone to hit him.

'No. Sorry. I thought ...' he seemed slightly at a loss momentarily. 'You went very white. I thought you were going to faint.'

'I probably am,' I retorted, angry that there seemed to be something actually wrong with me. After all, I had gone through

1

with the check-up to make sure that there *wasn't* something wrong with me. It was a safeguard, a check. It was never supposed to result in them finding something. 'I don't understand what you're telling me.'

The consultant started to explain about malignant tumours, abnormal cell growth, the tests he had run etc. and I listened calmly. Then, suddenly, during his patient, almost child-like explanation, a thought suddenly dawned on me. My stomach flipped, my heart pounded and I gasped with the shock of realisation.

'Are you saying I've got breast cancer?' I gasped.

'We *think* you've got breast cancer,' he amended, and began explaining again about the biopsy test he'd just performed, the degrees of certainty of a correct diagnosis so far. I sat forward, hunched over, my legs crossed, my hands clasped. I kept squeezing one hand with the other, as it was the only sensation or feeling that seemed to penetrate my senses and bring me back to the present.

'Breast cancer. They think I have breast cancer. I'm dying. I have a terminal illness. Looking at the outside of me, you could never tell. When I put my make-up on this morning, I didn't look like a woman with a terminal illness. But the inside paints a totally opposite picture.' These thoughts ran round my brain as the consultant carried on talking.

One of the women stepped forward as the consultant introduced her. She was the Breast Care Counsellor. I smiled automatically as we were introduced, and became aware that everyone was talking to me like I was a toddler. My world was suddenly made up of Noddy-language and simple sentence structures. But it was the only language I was capable of understanding. I felt punch-drunk.

The consultant said that this Counsellor was going to look after me, take me to a room where I could phone... a husband? Mother? Sister? I supplied the word 'husband' for him, and allowed myself to be led out of the consulting room, past the waiting room where I had sat only twenty minutes earlier in blissful ignorance of the time-bomb that was ticking away inside me.

Only twenty minutes. The earth had just cataclysmically stopped spinning, and time had slowed down to almost a standstill – yet twenty whole minutes had passed by. All the other twenty minuteses of the day had been so uneventful. Yet this twenty minutes was a twenty minutes I would play over and over again in my brain for the next couple of years.

And that is how my story begins. All the other events in my life led me to this point, and this moment suddenly changed my whole future landscape. Suddenly, instead of living life with the full expectation of reaching my guaranteed three score years and ten, it looked as though I was going to have to fight to get much past the halfway point. Instead of slaving away today to save for my retirement, it seemed that I didn't need to bother. Instead of not having time for my nearest, dearest and the things in life I most valued, it looked as though I had better enjoy them today because I might not have a chance in the future.

'Surely it can't be that much of a shock,' I hear you saying, 'considering you took yourself off to the doctor in the first place. You must have suspected something. Something must have been wrong. Surely you'd mentally prepared for this possibility?'

No. I hadn't. And let me explain why… because I had never felt a lump in my breast. I went to the doctor because I'd had a pain in my breast that came and went over the course of the six months leading up to this moment. But cancer is known as the Silent Killer. That's because in the early stages, it is rarely – if ever – accompanied by any pain. The entire medical team that treated me over the next eight months all said exactly the same. So I came to consider myself lucky that I had pain, as the location of the lump was such that I would not have felt it until it was very advanced. So was it a guardian angel watching over me? In fact, as I lay in hospital a week later, I reassured myself that this breast cancer wasn't going to kill me because I was being watched over. My oncologist, living in the real world, rationalised the pain as the tumour occasionally touching a nerve – which certainly sounds more reasonable. But reason deserted me in those first few months, and I grasped at anything, scientific or mythical, to convince myself that I would make a full recovery.

Let me just go back a couple of months. In January 2000, after an inauspicious start to the new millennium, I took myself off to see my GP. She wasn't unduly worried, saying that while she could feel a slight thickening of the tissue behind my nipple, it certainly didn't feel like a lump – certainly not the 2cm lump it later turned out to be. But she is a thorough and conscientious doctor, and sent me off for an ultrasound at Kingston Hospital. Thank you, Dr Boxer.

I got the appointment letter on the Thursday evening, though I didn't even see it until the Friday morning, as I had been too tired to bother looking at the post the night before. On the Friday morning I quickly ripped open the previous day's post.

'They don't give you much notice,' I said to my husband Colin, slapping the paper down on the dining room table. He looked briefly at it as he packed his bag ready for work.

'Cancel it,' he shrugged, trying to find some papers he'd left on the dining table a few weeks ago. His wife *always* moved things, because, as she always said, a dining table is for dining, not storing papers. But we were so cramped for space in this house, we didn't have anywhere to put papers.

'I will,' I said, folding the letter and putting it into my bag, and carried on rushing around getting ready for work.

Colin was about to walk out of the door, when he paused for a moment. 'If you do end up going, do you want me to be there?' he asked.

'Where? Oh the hospital? Whatever for?' I said absently, my mind on work. 'This is only routine. I'm not worried about it.'

'That's fine. Give me a call if you change your mind. Bye!' said Colin and left. I decided I'd also make a hasty departure in order to ring the clinic before going into my nine o'clock meeting. I had a jampacked day, as I was overseeing our company's name change – all stationery, answering machine etc, and D-day was Monday. We had *a lot* to get through to ensure it actually happened. I hastily kissed the kids goodbye before leaping into the car and driving to the other side of Kingston where my office was – only a twenty minute walk from home, but for me every second counted.

Friday 18th May, 9am

I charged up to my desk – I had long ago lost the art of walking – and flung bags and coats down. My two colleagues who sat in the same area as me were away for the day, so I had a modicum of privacy to make my call, which I decided to do first before I clean forgot about it.

'Hi. I got a letter last night advising my of an appointment at eleven o'clock this morning,' I said irritably – I really had too much to do to have to worry about *this*. 'It's very short notice, and a bit inconvenient.'

'Well, we try to see people in the week we get the letter from their GP,' the woman said, surprised that someone was complaining about the speed of their fast response. This was the NHS after all! 'We only do the clinic on Fridays, so if you can't make today we can do next Friday.'

'I'm away next week – it's half term.'

'The Friday after?'

I was momentarily tempted but two weeks away was another two weeks, and Dr Boxer had found something. And I knew full well that in two weeks time I would have yet another heavy workload or work emergency that would be equally critical, and I would put the appointment off again, and again. I paused for a second, then made a decision. 'No, I'll come today,' I said decisively, looking at my watch. My first meeting was starting now, so I confirmed my attendance at the clinic for eleven, and rang off.

My meeting went on for an hour, and at the end I rushed back to my desk and picked up my bag and coat. Hannah, the team secretary, came upstairs and looked questioningly at me.

'Have you got another meeting?' she said, not having seen it in my diary.

'Yeah – at the hospital actually. I'm going for a screening – nothing important – just… because… um… huh! They want to look at my breasts! I don't know when I'll be back. I may be some time,' I said, before rushing off. Wasn't it Captain Oates who famously said that, I reflected later on that evening?

> *Lesson learned:*
> **Don't put off having a check up.**

I pause in my reflections to acknowledge my general state of mind and lifestyle up to this point – how blissfully unaware I was, how preoccupied I was with all the trivial issues in my life that seemed so utterly important. Yet later on that evening, all of these really important things had faded to insignificance. The night hours ticked by as I allowed shock to absorb me, my eyes swollen from crying, as I gazed at the leaflets and pamphlets which described the known causes and subsequent treatments for breast cancer. I picked up the Macmillan booklet about breast cancer, and started flicking through it again but while my eyes read, my mind did not acknowledge. I put it down again, mentally reviewing the day's events, as though left brain was still trying to communicate the facts through to right brain; but each time I ran through that five minutes in the hospital when the consultant surgeon advised me the lump was malignant, my right brain heard the news afresh each time, and delivered a fresh sense of shock to my body.

Friday 18*th* February, 11am

When I arrived at the hospital earlier that day I had wisely, but without any sense of premonition, loaded up the parking meter to 6pm that evening, and reported to reception. A nurse handed me a huge bin bag and an outsize blue cotton bathrobe and told me to change then sit back down again. For the next hour I alternately waited, had an ultrasound, waited again, had a mammogram, then sat down to wait again. On the ultrasound screen I had seen a huge dark shadow on the screen, but while I knew it was a lump I had not for a second suspected it would be a malignant lump. After all, the odds were stacked against my having breast cancer as I was not in the high risk category by any stretch of the imagination.

As the nurse handed the notes to me, I was about to say something offhand but saw the kindly look in her eyes, and the first sense of doubt began. I went back upstairs, whereupon I was instructed to lie on the bed and the consultant surgeon, without warning, did a fine needle test that scratched and hurt momentarily. I put this test down to thoroughness, and was still not alarmed.

The nurse told me calmly that they were just going to run some tests to be on the safe side, which would take a couple of hours. I could wait in the restaurant beside the Maternity Wing, and come back in around two hours.

Friday 18th February, 1pm

I obediently went off. As I sat down to eat some lunch – a sausage roll – those first feelings of doubt were beginning to affect me. The sausage roll tasted of cardboard, however much ketchup I doused it in. Thoughts of breast cancer hovered at the edge of my mind, making my eyes prick with tears of fear and a lump rise in my throat. I rang Colin, trying to keep the panic out of my voice, but he heard it.

'I'll come down,' he said, hoping he could cancel his older brother who was travelling up from Taunton for a five o'clock meeting.

'No. Don't,' I said quickly.

'Why not?' Colin asked, surprised.

I paused, then said honestly, 'Because, if we treat it like it might be serious, then it might be serious. Let's carry on assuming this is nothing.' I said. 'I'm sure they're just erring on the side of caution.'

Colin agreed reluctantly. 'Okay. But let me know the minute they give you the results.'

I promised him I would, and rang off. The practical side of me recalled that I'd been mid-project when I left the office, and that it would be wise to deal with an outstanding issue. I phoned a colleague, Jo, and briefed her on some work, then told her what was going on. Jo was horrified, and I found myself reassuring her, saying that I was sure it was nothing, that after all, I was only 35 – not a high risk category age – and there was no history of breast cancer in my family. I said I'd call back later.

I abandoned my sausage roll and decided to just sit in the waiting room. I had brought some work with me, and I felt more comfortable cocooned there, close to the medical team who would surely let me know at the first possible opportunity that everything was fine. Every now and again, the door would open but they would call in another woman. Some came out smiling, others with neutral expressions. One or two were frowning. But nobody was weeping in shock at their diagnosis. Each time I looked up, my heart pounded momentarily, then it subsided again as my name was not called.

Friday 18th February, 2.30pm

Time started to slow down with each minute that passed, and a sense of deadened sound began to invade my recollection of the sequence of events – the sound I associate with the moment they told me my father had died. Thud, thud, thud… Was it my heart slowing down as I dealt with the shock? Or the fact that both times I have heard chronically bad news, I have held my breath in order to let my mind and body absorb it totally?

Friday 18th February, 4pm

Liz, the breast care nurse, sat down opposite me, putting a cup of water down in front of me and moving the box of tissues closer.

'Do you want to ask any questions?' she asked gently.

'Am I going to die?' I asked simply.

'Not necessarily, and certainly not imminently. We believe we have found it fairly early, and the prognosis is generally very good nowadays,' she replied. While this should have sounded good and positive, all I heard was the lack of certainty… just the provisos, the caveats.

'Have you got children?' Liz asked.

'Yes,' I said in a strangled voice. I was trying not to think of the children as it would make me cry too much.

'Are you going to tell them?' Liz asked.

I wished she would shut up about my children. 'Tell them? They're five and four. What do you tell them? What have I *got* to tell them? That mummy's got an illness that could kill me…!' I shouted, then burst into noisy sobs. Liz let me cry for a while, relieved that I had broken down that first wall of emotion. She said later that she'd found my earlier calm control and acceptance more worrying than the hysteria of her other patients who'd gone howling down the corridor.

Fifteen minutes later Colin was being shown into the bare office where I sat at an unused desk, huddled up, white-faced, red-eyed and clutching several balls of tissue in my tightly closed fists. He saw immediately how I was trying to hold it all together, to remain in control. He hugged me, but I felt drained and empty. Emotionless. I just started talking to him about practicalities.

'I'm just trying to get PPP to send a claim form through so I can get the surgery to sign it tonight before they close for the weekend,' I said, and went on to explain what the doctor had said, what he planned to do, when he wanted to operate and just how much he was aiming to remove when he operated. All my coping skills suddenly put in an appearance as I started going into Organisational Overdrive.

'Right. You're not having a mastectomy,' Colin repeated, as though trying to get his brain to understand it. He stood in the middle of the room, trying to take in all the facts.

'We try to conserve as much of the breast as possible nowadays,' said Liz.

'Where's the consultant?' he asked, wanting to speak to the man who'd just brought such awful news into their lives. Mr Wintry walked in at that moment, and introduced himself.

Colin fired off some questions, and Mr Wintry answered them as perfunctorily as he had his patient's. They were the same questions, and the same answers. After half an hour Mr Wintry made a move to leave, saying he would wait for our call.

'Just get rid of the cancer and make sure my wife lives, please,' said Colin. 'She's the only one I've got, and the only one I want,' he added helplessly, sitting down beside me and pulling me towards him. I slumped against him as Mr Wintry and Liz discreetly left the room.

Friday 18th February, 5.15pm

On the way home, an hour later, Colin phoned his mother, Rita, who was looking after the children. He told her what had happened so we didn't have to go into complex explanations in front of the children as to why we were arriving home together. We walked in and I kissed my children hello, trying to look normal. They were drawing pictures and didn't notice anything untoward, not realising the cataclysm that was happening around them. Or so I thought.

'I've drawn a picture of you,' said my son, Eliot, ten minutes later. This was an amazing enough feat in itself, as Eliot didn't ever draw. I took the picture and saw he had drawn a picture of me with tears pouring down my face.

'Oh? Have I hurt myself?' I asked, my throat choking with emotion.

'No. You're sad,' he said simply. I always suspected he was a sensitive little boy despite his boisterous attitude to life, but now I wondered whether he was actually psychic.

'Well, draw me with a smiley face on the other side of the paper, to show that I get happy again after my sadness,' I said. He took it back obligingly.

Friday 18th February, 6pm

I went upstairs to call mother and my sister. I couldn't ring my brothers in Hong Kong as it would be four o'clock in the morning for them. I tried my mother first, at the school where she worked. A colleague, Mike Fanya, answered.

'Hi, is Rosie there?' I asked, and was advised that she had left half an hour earlier. He asked if everything was alright and I tried to say everything was fine. I added that he might want to call mum a little bit later – she might want someone to talk to. I tried mum's house. No answer. Obviously still en route. I tried her mobile number, and finally she answered.

'Hiya,' I said trying to sound light. 'Where are you?'

'In Homebase buying a bathmat,' said my mother, wondering why I was calling at this time on a Friday evening.

'Oh, okay. I was just phoning for a chat. When will you be home?'

'In about half an hour,' said my mother, doubt instinctively gnawing at her heart as she put the bathmat down, deciding to buy it another day. Joanna *never* rang for a chat on a Friday at six o'clock… she was rarely even home at that time, let alone making leisurely phone calls. Mother's instinct told her something was terribly wrong, and that she should just get home. 'I'll call you when I get there.'

'Okay. Speak to you later.' I rang off. Rose ran out of the store and drove home like the clappers, wondering all the way what could have happened.

Next I rang my sister. 'Hi,' I said when Kate answered.

'Hi,' Kate said cheerily down the phone. 'I can't stop for long, as I've just put the kids to bed and am about to start dinner.'

'That's okay. I'm not in the mood for a long chat,' I said. 'I've just had some bad news, very bad news.'

'Oh no, what?' Kate sounded panicky immediately.

'You know I mentioned a week or two ago that I went to the doctor about a "not-lump".'

'Oh no, what?' Kate repeated.

'It's malignant.'

'Oh no!' Kate whispered in horror. I remained silent, trying to find my voice again. 'When did you find out?' Kate asked.

'Just now,' I muttered, straining to keep control. 'I mean, a couple of hours ago.'

'What have they said about it?' Kate asked, trying to get her brain round the shock of it.

'Firstly that the prognosis is fairly good nowadays.' I got a grip on myself, and started trying to reassure my sister. I told Kate in detail what had happened that day, recounting it stage by stage as though telling myself for the first time, and my voice felt muffled as though I was speaking from a long way away.

'I just can't believe it.' Kate said for the fourth time and told me about somebody nearby who'd just had cancer. I felt overwhelmingly tired and needed some more time to think again. For me there was nothing further to say about the subject, and Kate was too stunned to speak.

'I'm waiting for mum to call me back. I haven't told her yet. I may try to call you later,' I said, then suggested we speak again the next day. We rang off, and the ensuing silence echoed in my brain as I looked round the bedroom, looking for some kind of lifeboat, but there was nothing.

My mother called back ten minutes later. 'Hello,' she said, and jumped right in. 'What's up?'

I told her firstly that I'd been to the hospital that day, as my mother didn't even know that much as yet, and then told her the diagnosis, quickly followed by all the reassurances about good prognoses, finding it early, imminent operation etcetera.

'For once you've silenced me,' Rose said, putting her hand up to her forehead as though to still her whirling mind. Her four children had delivered many surprising pieces of news to her over the years – pregnancies, marriages, global travel plans, emigration plans, ill health, broken bones, arguments whatever – and she had taken them all in her stride, never fazed by any of them. She'd always had the right words of congratulations or sympathy, condolences or advice, and had never yet felt lost for words. But now words failed her.

'I think it's silenced me as well,' I said. 'Rare for the both of us.'

Mum then asked me loads of questions about what, and how, and where, and how bad, and since when. I answered what I could, until finally I said I was going to soak in the bath, and we both hung up. Rose stared dry-eyed for a moment at the phone before the floodgates opened and she cried, and cried, and cried.

Rita offered to stay, to look after the children, but Colin and I needed some time alone. She didn't say very much to me, but I knew that was out of sensitivity and shock. After she left, I put the children to bed while Colin made some phone calls from the conservatory. I sat down on the sofa, staring wide-eyed at the television with the sound off. I didn't want to hear anything. Colin came in and sat down beside me, and we both just sat there in mutual shock, occasionally breaking the silence to go over things the surgeon had said, to try and understand what was going on, talking over the 'what if's...?' What if the cancer had gone to the lymph nodes? What if I needed radiotherapy? Or chemotherapy? What if...? Several hours passed in this vein.

'We have choices,' Colin said. 'Mr Wintry said we have choices, but let's take it all one step at a time.'

The phone rang beside me, and I turned my head slowly to look at it before picking it up. It was my mother.

'How are you?'

'I don't know. I'm trying to work that out.'

'I was just ringing to suggest that I come up tomorrow morning early and take the children from you. I should have thought of it earlier, before they went to bed,' said Rose, desperate to do something to help and wanting to see her daughter.

'Thanks.'

'Do you want to talk?' my mother said, knowing I was not really listening.

'I've got nothing to say,' I said, too stunned to speak.

'Have you got information to read? Or a counsellor you can speak to tonight?'

'I've got some booklets… from Cancer Bacup… and the Macmillan nurses.'

'And phone numbers for a counsellor?' she persisted.

'Yes.' I looked at Liz's card, with no intention of calling her. I needed time to think and read, not talk. I had to work out my questions first.

'And will you call her?'

'If I need to.'

'Call me if you want to discuss anything. And tell Colin to call me if he wants to talk.'

'Thanks. I think I just need to think. I need to read the books they gave me.'

'Any time during the night… just call me. I want to be here for you.'

'I know.'

There was a silence down the line, my mother reluctant to hang up. She would have preferred to keep the line open all night, just sitting there with the phone held up to her ear in case I suddenly wanted to talk about my feelings or ask questions that neither of us could answer but we could analyse together.

'I'm going to read these booklets.' I said finally. 'And don't worry, Mum. I have a very long lifeline.'

'We're a family with very long lives.' Mum grasped at the straw immediately – I suspect more to reassure me than any real belief on her part. 'Grandad had bladder cancer nearly thirty years ago, and he's ninety-four this year.'

'Absolutely. And they say I've found this early,' I agreed.

'And treatments get better the whole time.'

'Absolutely,' I said. We were both desperately searching for reassurances.

'Call me any time of the night if you want to talk.'

'I will.' And we hung up again.

Friday 18th February, 10pm

That evening went on forever. ten, 10.01, 10.02… it ticked by so slowly. Too early to go to bed, too much to think about to watch television, too little knowledge to discuss, too much fear to voice out loud. We spent the evening sometimes sitting wild-eyed on the sofa, sometimes wandering from room to room as though looking for peace of mind, which we didn't find. At some point, Colin phoned my boss, Dave, to tell him what was happening. I was too far beyond speech, and not able to voice my devastating news to anyone other than my family, in case I cracked and became hysterical. Colin emerged from the conservatory red-eyed but I didn't ask about their conversation.

He told me some of it. 'Apparently one of the directors in your sister company has just been through this – his wife Lesley had breast cancer last year. Dave's suggested you phone her if you want to, and he's given me the number.' He went on to discuss some technical medical developments in breast cancer care that Dave also knew about, but it went over my head.

Friday 18th February, 11pm

Finally Colin and I decided to go to bed. We went upstairs, crawling under the covers and clinging onto each other as though the bed was a life raft. But it wasn't. After lying there wide awake for an hour, I wriggled out of Colin's arms and got out of bed. Colin asked me if I was alright, and I said I was going downstairs.

'Do you want me to come down as well?' he asked.

'I want to be alone for a while. I need to think,' I said, knowing he would understand.

'Okay,' he said, and I left him staring sleeplessly into the darkness.

I picked up one of the booklets and started to read. Normally I scanned pages, skimming down through the centre of the page, my eyes picking out key sentences and paragraphs, but now I read each word, from the beginning of the line to the end, line by line to the end of each page as though hoping that some clue or answer would clarify the confusion in my brain. I didn't know what clue or answer I was looking for, but something, something that would make me understand what was happening, why, and where it was going.

In fact, none of the listed reasons applied to me. No family members had had breast or other linked cancers. *High risk age is over 55 years...* '*I'm only thirty-five!*' I mentally screamed at the book. Nobody in my family has had breast cancer, I said mentally to the next point. *Postponing pregnancy...* I was just thirty when I'd given birth to Grace, and I had read recently that the national average for first births was now thirty years of age. So again, no. Next point: breast-feeding mothers have a lower risk of developing breast cancer. I'd breast-fed my children briefly before moving onto bottles in order to return to work. *Starting your periods early...* no – I was thirteen which, at that time, was the national average

Next... *taking the Pill.* I had always been hopeless at remembering to take it and Colin had always been reluctant for me to be on the Pill as he didn't like the thought of tablets messing around with one's natural state. *Being seriously overweight...* No, thank you very much. I had been size ten up to my mid-twenties, then had fluctuated between sizes twelve and fourteen over the last six years, during my two pregnancies. *Drinking and smoking* increase the chances. Well, certainly I had drunk plenty enough alcohol since my teens, but no one could call that excessive. I was the same as any other woman enjoying a good social life. And I had smoked socially for eight or so years, but given up when I met Colin. So again, while these may have been contributory factors, my current condition certainly couldn't be ascribed directly to them.

Last point... *starting the menopause early, or taking hormone replacement therapy*. Again, neither applied *because I'm only thirty-five*, I mentally shouted again at the book. *I'm thirty-five with two young children, and too young to die.* And I burst into tears afresh.

Friday 18th February, midnight

When I dried my eyes half an hour later, I picked the book up again and continued reading the section on the Symptoms of Breast Cancer, searching for signals and signs that I had clearly missed.

But no. I had not had any of the classic symptoms. There had been the pain in the breast, but the book denied that this was a symptom, and some types of benign lumps are painful anyway. No hints. No clues. Nothing that could have forewarned me. It made the shock worse. I hadn't even suspected anything.

I threw the book across the room for being wrong. I stared angrily at it as it landed by the armchair. Apart from a dull ache, I'd never had any symptoms, no lumps, nothing.

I stood up, and poured myself a small brandy, gulping down the first shot. It burned the back of my throat, and felt good, jolting me into a sense of reality and reminding me I was still alive.

That thought shook me... I was still alive. Of course! I was actually still alive. I smiled with relief... I was actually still alive, I repeated to myself. I wasn't hit by a truck today. I wasn't run over or killed in a car crash. I'd had some bad news, that's all.

I think it was at this point I began to turn the corner. Not a bad distance to travel in twelve hours. It dawned on me that I had learned something important that was likely to see me through this new journey I had embarked upon – that where there's life, there's hope. This realisation was the first important lesson on the long road back to health.

> ## Lesson learned:
> ## Where there's life, there's hope.

February 19th 2000, 1am

I felt re-energised by this new realisation, and decided that positive action was called for. I needed to understand what this illness was. I needed more information. I needed to keep pumping information in until I reached some level of comprehension about what was going to happen, what I might expect, and what I could do to help myself. I retrieved the discarded booklet and carried on reading.

The Stages of Breast cancer:
- *Ductal carcinoma in situ: when the cancer cells are completely contained within the ducts, and have not spread into the surrounding breast tissue. This is almost always completely cured.*
- *Stage one tumours: measure less than 2 cm, the lymph glands are not affected and there are no signs that it has spread elsewhere in the body.*
- *Stage two tumours: measure between 2 and 5 cm, or the lymph glands in the armpit are affected, or both, but there are no signs that it has spread further.*
- *Stage three tumours: larger than 5cm, lymph glands usually affected but there are no signs of further spread*
- *Stage four tumour: of any size, the lymph glands are usually affected and the cancer has spread to other parts of the body. This is secondary breast cancer.*

I read word by word as though studying for an exam. I was sure that by tomorrow, I would indeed be able to sit an exam on this subject. The surgeon had said mine was a 2 cm lump, and that made it early Stage 2 and that the lymph nodes might well be affected. *This stage of cancer is usually treated with surgery and radiotherapy, and possibly chemotherapy.* I sighed heavily.

I began to plough through the pages of *Coping with Surgery* and *Living with Breast Surgery.* Radiotherapy, chemotherapy… I paused to have a quick read over that section. It appeared there were many ways they could administer chemotherapy, different types of chemotherapy and different reactions to it. I read but did not absorb much of it. I knew, as with the rest of the population, that chemotherapy caused your hair to fall out, and chronic tiredness and sickness. I had absorbed so much tonight, and my first priority was surgery rather than chemotherapy, so I skimmed over this section, deciding to come back to it at a later date.

I skimmed through a further ten pages, until I reached a page headed *Your Feelings,* under which there was a bold sub-heading *Shock and Disbelief.* Oh yes, plenty of shock and disbelief, and I wasn't surprised to read *'the need for repetition is a common reaction to shock'*. My eyes went back to the top of the page in order to read the section properly.

Your Feelings:
• Shock and disbelief – 'I can't believe it, it just can't be true.'
You may feel numb, unable to believe what is happening and unable to express any emotion. You may be able to only absorb small pieces of information, and need to keep asking the same questions over and over again, and have the answers told to you simply and repeatedly.

• Fear and uncertainty – 'Am I going to die? Will I be in pain?'
Cancer is a frightening word, surrounded by many fears and myths. In fact, many cancers nowadays, including breast cancer, are curable if caught at any early stage. Even later stage cancers can be controlled for years with modern treatments, with patients living almost normal lives. Many people elect to sort out their affairs upon diagnosis, which provides peace of mind and this is always helpful.
Some people do not experience pain, and for those who do, modern drugs, radiotherapy and nerve blocks can ease the pain.
Uncertainty about the future can cause a lot of tension, but fears are invariably worse than the reality. Gaining knowledge about your illness can be reassuring, and discussing this with your family and friends can help relieve the tension of unnecessary worry.

• Denial – 'There's nothing really wrong with me.'
Some people prefer to not discuss their illness, and you should say to people around you that you would prefer not to talk about it, at least for the time being. Sometimes it is the other way around, with family or friends who are denying your illness, possibly thinking that changing the subject will play down your anxieties, and they can appear to ignore the fact that you have cancer. Let them know that it will help you if you can talk to them about your illness.

• Anger – 'Why me of all people? And why right now?' Anger can hide feelings such as fear or sadness, and you may vent this anger on those close to you, and on the doctors and nurses who are caring for you. Sometimes

your anger may upset those around you, and you will need to tell them that your anger is about your illness and not really directed at them.

• Blame and guilt – 'If I hadn't... this would never have happened.'
You may try to find reasons why this should have happened to you, as often we feel better when we understand why something has happened, and this can result in you blaming yourself. However, doctors rarely know exactly what has caused an individual's cancer, and there is therefore no reason for you to blame yourself.

• Resentment – 'It's alright for you, you don't have to put up with this.'
You may feel resentful and miserable because you have cancer while everyone else is well. You can resent the changes it makes to your life during treatment, and sometimes relatives will also resent the impact it has on their lives. However, don't bottle it up, as this exacerbates a problem and makes everyone feel angry and guilty.

• Withdrawal and isolation – 'Leave me alone!'
There may be times during your illness or treatment that you need to be left alone to sort out your thoughts and emotions. This can be tough on family and friends who want to help you through this difficult time, and you may need to reassure them that you will involve them when you are ready. Depression can stop you wanting to talk, and you may need to discuss this with your GP, who can help you.

• Learning to cope
After any treatment for cancer, it can take a long time to come to terms with your emotions. Not only do you have to cope with the knowledge that you have cancer, but also the physical effects of the treatment. You need to relax in order to recover, and only do as much as you feel you can.

I read the contents of each paragraph, then stared at the walls trying to feel which of these feelings I was experiencing the most. But such a large part of me felt numb that I couldn't sense anything... obviously Shock & Disbelief. I wondered if I would go through the list of feelings before reaching the Learning to Cope.

Friday 19ᵗʰ February, 4am

And how would my children cope?

Bang! The children were in my head. I had fought so hard to keep my thoughts from straying to them, as I knew this was the bit that was going to crucify me. The tears came suddenly, and flowed fast. I could picture their trusting little faces, and feel their hearts breaking if anything happened to me. I was their life. I knew what it was like to lose a parent. I was eleven when my father died and I knew too well and too clearly the hole it leaves in your life, the pain and the confusion. They would have to learn how to live with that empty hollowness that the death of a parent leaves in the core of you, the pain of wanting to talk to someone who's no longer there, the longing to hold you and feeling the coldness in the absence of the hug; they would have to deal with the confusion of why their mummy had to die, the bewilderment of life itself, all the while wanting mummy's advice on day to day problems; they would have to cope with feeling unloved and lacking security.

It was with these thoughts whirling through my mind that I cried myself to sleep, just as dawn was breaking outside.

Source: Cancer Bacup 'Understanding Cancer of the Breast'

Further reading "What is Cancer"
on the website www.careerkidsandbreastcancer.com

Chapter Two
Being the bearer of bad news

Saturday 19th February, 9am

I woke up on the sofa, having slept fitfully; I had woken up every fifteen minutes or so, sweating and my mind racing. Each time I woke up, I recalled the fact that I had just been diagnosed with cancer, and my stomach would flip and my heart start pounding. Now it was morning and life still felt unreal. My stomach was still churning and my eyes felt dry and itchy from crying all night. On the floor beside the sofa was an A4 page with reams of questions I wanted answers to; and my head was bursting with all the information I had learned about breast cancer within an incredibly short space of time.

The children came downstairs and were surprised to see me sitting on the edge of the sofa already. I smiled at them, feeling dizzy with lack of sleep, and muttered something about a bath. I climbed the stairs on auto-pilot, but on reaching the bathroom I decided I could not be bothered to run myself a bath. I walked into the bedroom, where Colin was lying on his back, eyes wide open.

'Alright?' he said.

'I think so,' I said, opening the wardrobe doors and standing uselessly in front of my clothes. None of them appealed, I decided. I couldn't be bothered to think about what to wear, and anyway, I was still dressed from yesterday, so what the hell.

'Come here,' said Colin. I complied, and lay back down beside him again. 'Don't shut me out. Tell me what you're thinking.'

'It goes something like *arghhhhhhhhhhhhhhhh*,' I said, flapping my hands in the air round my head. Colin laughed with relief that I hadn't lost my humour.

'What else?' he said.

'I'll tell you when I know.'

'Don't shut me out.' he repeated. I promised I wouldn't, then got up restlessly and went back downstairs.

In the kitchen, I opened up the fridge, then the food cupboards, but decided against eating any breakfast because it would still taste of cardboard. Instead I opted for a coffee. I flicked the kettle on and wandered over to the front door to collect the newspaper.

The headlines were announcing that the internet boom bubble had burst, that stocks and shares were plummeting – none of which seemed important, although I had been following the rise and launch of Lastminute.com and, up until yesterday, had been interested in the outcome. But now all that had suddenly become unimportant.

I put the newspaper down, and floated round the downstairs of the house like a lost soul. What? What could I do? I needed someone to talk to, someone who would not offer sympathy but some kind of insight, some answers… But who the hell would that be? Who could put my mind at rest? If the surgeon, with his many years experience in breast cancer, couldn't, then where did that leave my army of family and friends?

First and foremost, I actually needed to rearrange my week as suddenly all my plans had been cast asunder. It was half term, and I had been planning to take the latter half of the week off work to go and visit my close friend, Miranda, down in the West country. However, I would clearly not be going into work now, or to Dorset. Instead I would be going into hospital. The children could go to my mother's for a few days.

I also wanted to talk to both my brothers – it would be early evening in Hong Kong, which was probably a good time to try. I tried them both, but neither was in. I left messages just saying that I was trying to call would try again over the weekend – enough to let them know I specifically wanted to chat but not enough to alarm them. Then I decided I would ring Miranda, to cancel my visit. She answered sleepily, and I realised that it was still only 9am.

'Sorry, I've called a bit early, haven't I?' I apologised meekly. Miranda hated mornings.

'No. It's alright.' Miranda tucked the phone between her ear and shoulder, and snuggled back under the covers. 'I hope you're not phoning to cancel.'

'I am, but before you say anything,' I said quickly, so she didn't make a fuss then feel guilty after I'd told her why, 'I've had some bad news. I've got to go into hospital this week.'

'Oh no.' Miranda sounded vaguely alarmed. 'Why?'

'I have to have a lump removed from my breast,' I said, wondering if this way of telling people was better than just baldly coming out with the 'I've Got Breast Cancer' statement.

'You poor thing. It's not, er, what's the word…?' Miranda had difficulty with big words. 'It's not a bad lump, is it?'

I breathed in. 'Yes. It is malignant.' Tears stung my eyes again. 'It's breast cancer.'

'No! I don't believe it!' Miranda sat up, shocked. 'Jo! What have they said to you?'

'That I've found it fairly early and the prognosis is quite good. They don't know if it's gone to my lymph nodes yet, but don't believe it's gone anywhere else beyond that.' I rattled off what was to become a stock-in-trade reassurance. We talked for a while longer and Miranda said she would come up and visit as soon as I wanted her to.

After hanging up, I sat back heavily. It was just as tough telling people as being told the news yourself, if not worse. At least hearing the news yourself you are managing your own reactions, whereas when you tell people your bad news you then need to cope with their reactions, trying to re-lighten the atmosphere after delivering such bad news. I tried to imagine how I would feel had it been the other way round, if Miranda had just called me and said that she had cancer. I would be lost for words, full of 'I don't believe it' and 'how awful', then trying to find something comforting or reassuring, or at the very least helpful.

The word 'cancer' strikes fear into people's hearts as it has such ominous and final connotations. Cancer is such a big word, a word that everyone knows and fears. And why? Because one thing we all know about cancer is that it is a death sentence, ultimately. And beyond this one big and scary piece of information, none of us knows terribly much. We all know people who have suffered and died from cancer, much as we all know people who have suffered and recovered from cancer. But do we really believe they have totally recovered? Or do we believe they are merely mid-process, in remission or some kind of limbo where they are waiting to see when it returns?

I realised that, up until yesterday, this is what I had believed. My father had died from lung cancer and a close friend of Colin's had died a year earlier from throat cancer after a three-year battle. While my father's death was very quick following diagnosis, although that was largely because he had avoided seeing a doctor for so long, which meant the cancer was very advanced by the time it was diagnosed. Also, that was twenty-five years ago, when treatments were far less sophisticated than today.

Colin's friend, Ray, who'd died from throat cancer, had also discovered his condition when it was fairly advanced. He had undergone extensive surgery, and there had been times since his surgery when he'd looked really quite well. He had been very optimistic about his chances, which had been slim from the start: a one in five chance of the cancer returning within the year, I seem to recall. But even when he'd looked well, I remembered my own difficulty with talking to him about it, trying to find the optimistic view as he discussed his health, because deep down I didn't feel optimistic for him at all. I believed, as with the rest of the nation, that cancer is cancer, and you die from it.

I remembered Ray's funeral. Colin had been a huge support to Celia, his widow, who had actually looked pretty together throughout the service. Colin and Ray's nephew had given such lovely and moving speeches that left many people in tears. I had found tears pouring down my face uncontrollably as Colin recalled some of the good times spent with Ray, and I was nearly on the floor when he said 'One thing that really pained me, and probably all of us here today, is that Ray did not want to die. He fought to the bitter end, and was so angry about his illness.' The woman next to me was well prepared with tissues, and had handed me a bundle as I started crying quite hard. It was only once they got outside that I saw the blank look in Celia's eyes that masked the pain, not only of today, but of the many months of helping Ray through his illness and preparing for his death.

I reached for the tissues now as the tears once again started to run down my face at the memory of Ray. And what do *I* think of death? I pondered. After all, I now have cancer. I am one of those people who have it. Why me? Because why not me! Why should I be any different from anyone else in this country that has a percentage chance of developing cancer. I am one of this nation's statistics, and therefore why not me? And what do I now think of cancer? Do I still believe today, as I did up until yesterday, that it is a one way street with some parking places to pause for a while, but ultimately heading to the big STOP sign at the end? Or do I believe that I have a chance here, that I may be able to turn off and take a much longer detour before I hit the end of the road?'

A paragraph from the MacMillan booklet I had read the night before referred to 'The Cancer Journey', and this popped into my mind now. The map of this journey showed key points in the process of cancer treatment, and the various exit points en route, some of which said 'cure', and one to the big exit point at the end following palliative care. It was similar to a motorway, with various junctions whereby you can leave or rejoin the motorway. Is this what cancer really is? Is it more like a motorway than just a one-way street with no turn-offs? Did I now believe that I could turn off this street?

I mulled this over now. Did I feel like I was dying? No. I certainly didn't feel like it was curtains for me. In fact, I felt relatively well – a bit tired, a bit headachy, but certainly nowhere near death. And where there's life, there's life, I reasoned to myself. I actually have a life to live, and while I have a life, I'll damn well live it – and work hard at trying to turn off this Cancer Journey motorway.

I suddenly felt strong, and breathed in deeply. Oxygen felt good. I was flooded with a positive feeling, and congratulated myself on this after – ooh, what was it? – only twenty hours into knowing I was facing treatment for breast cancer.

I went into the kitchen and made a piece of toast, while I was feeling strong and positive – before that dry mouth fear returned. I put some toast down in front of the children, who were already glued to Cartoon Network. So what? I sat down with them, and tried to watch it with them. But my mind started to wander again. What had triggered this in the beginning? What could I do to stop that trigger happening again?

11am

I picked up my discarded list of questions off the floor, and wrote that at the top as a priority question, wondering whether I should call the surgeon and confirm Wednesday. But I wasn't quite ready yet… I needed to speak to someone who would confirm that it was the right thing to do. After all, I felt like I was just accepting the first quote – which I never did when booking a builder, or finding a nanny. And if I always got at least three quotes and references for builders, and interviewed at least seven or eight nannies to look after my precious babies, then why on earth should I take the first quote from a surgeon who was going to put me to sleep and cut me open for such a potentially life-saving operation? After all, he'd better cut the whole tumour out properly the first time rather than leaving a bit in which carried on growing and spreading. I shuddered at this thought.

I wanted to seek a broader opinion, but who on earth did I go to for further quotes? After all, surgeons aren't exactly listed in the phone book under their surgery speciality. So how do you reach them? Through your doctor, but how do you know your doctor is sending you off to the right person? After all, there are dreadful stories in the newspapers about surgeons butchering and maiming people who have blindly trusted them; surgeons who had dreadful track records, yet whose references were never followed up when they were employed by the hospital. So how could I personally begin to get references on a surgeon?

Colin came downstairs as I was leafing through the Yellow Pages. 'What are you doing?' he asked.

'Looking up surgeons,' I said, slightly foolishly.

Colin nodded. 'Do you want a second opinion?'

'Maybe. But I just don't know where from?'

My head was beginning to ache, and I could feel myself working up again. How do you control that around you which is so utterly impossible to control? I suddenly didn't feel so strong. I felt overwhelmed and confused. My start point was to contact my GP, who of course would not be around on a Saturday so I would have to wait until Monday. Yet in the meantime, I needed to decide whether to go ahead with the surgery next week, and I really did not want this lump in my breast any longer than was absolutely necessary. Every day increased the possibility of it spreading to another part of my body, particularly under so much stress.

'*Ohhh!*' I groaned out loud and clutched my head in my hands. 'I need to phone someone, anyone, right now. I can't keep thinking. I just need someone to talk to, someone who's been there before.'

I reached for the number that Dave had given Colin last night, and dialled Lesley's number.

'Hi, my name's Joanna. I was…' I began when a woman answered the phone.

'Oh hello, Dave has already called me and said that you might call,' she said in a friendly, welcoming voice. 'I'm really pleased you have.'

'Is now a good time to chat, or would you rather I called back later?'

'No, now's perfect. The children are at various Saturday clubs with Peter as chauffeur. You only found out yesterday, didn't you?'

'Yeah, so I'm still pretty shocked, and agonising over a number of things…'

'It's a huge shock.' Lesley said comfortingly. 'I remember when I was told… I'd noticed the lump early in the summer, but kind of dismissed it; after all, I'm only forty-one now so I didn't really fit into the high risk category, and no-one in my family has had this. Anyway, what with the summer holidays etcetera, I decided to wait until they were over, then see a doctor. I finally went in mid-September, and couldn't believe it when they diagnosed the lump as malignant.'

'I'm similar, I suppose," I said as I went on to explain my story.

'Do they know what stage it is?' she asked finally.

'Early stage 2, as the lump's about 2cm.'

'I was mid stage 2, with a lump of around 3cm. So they did radio and chemotherapy first to shrink the tumour before doing a lumpectomy and removing the lymph nodes.'

'I'm the other way round; I have the lump removed next week, then they'll tell me whether I need the chemotherapy once they've checked the lymph nodes.'

'Well, you found it early, which is good.'

'Yes, they said they were surprised that I'd found it and consulted a doctor, because it wasn't even a lump… just a kind of change, but very subtle. How long ago were you diagnosed?'

'About two years ago, and in fact I just had my second year scan last week, and was given the all clear.'

'Oh that's great. And how was the treatment, all the radio and chemotherapy?'

'It was okay actually. Modern treatments are very good, and they just get better the whole time.'

'Were you very sick during chemotherapy?'

'No, not really, though I felt rather nauseous and very tired, particularly towards the end.'

'How many sessions did you have?'

'Six. Six is the standard for adjuvant therapy – which is the preventative course of treatment. You may have five or seven, but six is standard. Most of the other ladies I know had six.'

'And did you go bald?'

'Oh, completely!' she laughed. 'But that's nothing, it all grows back again – and I didn't have to shave for months!'

'You sound so well,' I said.

'Because I am. The prognosis is very good when you find it early. The only lady I know who has had a relapse did actually find it quite late.'

'And how old are your children?'

'They were seven and nine when I was diagnosed, so old enough to understand what was going on. And I was advised in the beginning to be honest with them, because my illness was a family issue. Children pick up tensions and problems very quickly, and if they feel there's a secret they are not party to, they can worry themselves into a real state. So I was honest, and told them – though obviously a very positive and optimistic version of my cancer and my treatment.'

'And did they cope quite well?'

'My seven-year-old son did, because he was younger and less given to pondering. My daughter worried more, but I kept talking to her about it and giving her loads of opportunities to voice her worries. It seemed to work, although it's so difficult to tell with children – particularly as they start puberty and become all secretive and silent with you!' Again, she chuckled. 'How old are yours?'

'Five and four, so I'm wondering how much I really need to tell them.'

'Well, you know your children better than anyone else so it's really up to you. But I would certainly suggest you tell them something.'

'I think you're right. Particularly as I have to go into hospital – let alone when I lose all my hair. I think they'll definitely realise something's up!'

'Yes. And your daughter may feel more sensitive about it than your son. Girls have a much bigger thing about hair at a very early age. It was one of the side-effects that really upset my daughter.'

'That's interesting to know.' I paused. 'Another thing I'm pondering – well in fact it's more than that – agonising over is the surgery. When you were diagnosed, did you get a number of opinions?'

'No, I just got the one opinion. Why?'

'Well, I'm probably just being silly—'

'—which is reasonable at this time,' interrupted Lesley, with a smile in her voice.

'Yeah… But how did you know that the surgeon and the oncologist you got were going to give you the best treatment?'

Lesley paused. 'Well I didn't really. I think I was so shocked that I just kind of went along with it all… but they were absolutely brilliant.'

'But it's a bit of a lottery, isn't it?'

'I guess it is, but you're in Kingston, which has a very good hospital, and you will probably be sent to one of the Centres of Excellence for your oncology - the chemo and radio etc."

'Oh, I see how it works. Then it's just a question of whether my surgeon is any good, and will he refer me to an oncologist at one of these centres?'

'Yes. To be honest, you're asking more questions at this stage than I was capable of. You do seem to be thinking very clearly. I was an emotional basket case,' she laughed at herself.

'Really?' I said surprised. 'I guess I just need to understand, and arrange everything around me properly before I get too emotional.' I realised as I spoke that I had mentally set aside four days for thinking, planning and organising, before I climbed into that hospital bed and caved in. 'Anyway, I really appreciate this chat… it's certainly helped just talking to you and making contact with someone else who has been through it. So far I've spoken to three experts, none of whom have actually had cancer, and it helps to hear you so positive and upbeat after all your treatment.'

'I hope it has helped. If there's anything else, do call me. You sound very calm and in control – which is good,' Lesley added.

'I feel in complete turmoil,' I admitted.

'Obviously you have great coping skills. Keep it up and do stay in touch, because I'd like to help.'

'I will. Definitely. And thanks.' We said goodbye and rang off. My optimism rose slightly again with the reassurance that Lesley sounded so well and so positive after all her treatment. I was also cheered by the fact that she thought I was coping well and was in control. I knew I wasn't in reality – but I was relieved that I seemed so to the outside world. It somehow spurred me on. While nothing had really altered about getting second opinions, I felt slightly more settled about Mr Wintry. Or maybe I just felt more settled, having spoken to Lesley. What a roller coaster of a ride this is going to be, I thought as I stood up and walked into the kitchen. One moment up, then down, then whizzed around 360° back down again.

I'd better hold on tight.

> *Lesson learned:*
> **Talk, Listen and Learn – for a problem shared is a problem halved.**

Midday

I made myself another cup of coffee and hovered in the kitchen for a moment, then I realised I was putting off making more phone calls. The next one had better be the surgeon, as I wanted to get this organised so I at least had one certainty in my life – however unpleasant that certainty was going to be.

'I'm going to phone Mr Wintry and go ahead with him,' I said to Colin as he hovered in the doorway, staring at me.

'You don't have to. We have choices,' he said, his voice hollow.

'I just want this lump removed,' I said, and he nodded. He walked back into the sitting room and plumped down on the sofa heavily, feeling useless and sick. He had been feeling sick since his wife had phoned him yesterday, and had not been able to eat or drink anything since then.

I called Mr Wintry, who was kind and reassuring but equally very matter-of-fact. I consulted my list of questions, asking him a couple of relevant ones, although I baulked at the one question I'd really have liked to ask – whether I could see his CV and references.

'Can you just remind me again of the process, because I think there was a lot I didn't hear yesterday evening after...' I trailed off.

'Yes,' he said, picking up the cue. 'We remove the lump, and possibly the lymph nodes; depending on what we find, we then recommend a course of follow-up treatment of radiotherapy, and possibly chemotherapy and Tamoxifen. But those are all choices at this stage, not specifics.'

'Do you administer all of that?'

'No, I'm the surgeon. I do the surgery, then recommend you to an oncologist who carries out all of the subsequent treatment.'

'And, out of interest, what would you say constitutes successful surgery?' I asked quickly, determined to get something out of this guy. He laughed, although I thought I could hear irritation in his laugh. 'You do ask unusual questions,' he began. 'But I'll answer. Successful surgery in this case is defined by removing not only the tumour, but also the wider area to ensure we have got all cancerous cells. It is additionally defined by the successful removal of the lymph nodes, which are difficult to remove as they are spread around under the arm.'

'I see. And how many operations of this type have you done?'

The penny obviously dropped with him at that point that he was actually being interviewed for his suitability to operate on me. 'Look, it is completely your right to get a second opinion if you don't trust mine…' he began defensively.

'I'm not asking these questions because of my "rights", and I don't doubt your diagnosis for a second although it would be my dearest wish that you were actually wrong. I just want to know who you are before you do surgery on me. I'm not trying to be antagonistic, or challenge your capabilities. In fact, I actually want to hear you boast about them. And surely, as a thinking man, you would do exactly the same, wouldn't you?' I said, knowing my bluntness had probably offended him – it frequently offended many people, but I couldn't help it. I wanted straight answers, so I asked straight questions.

Mr Wintry's tone softened slightly. 'Yes, I would. I have done more lumpectomies and mastectomies than I would ever have wished. Breast cancer is shockingly prevalent, and in younger and younger women, and nothing gives me greater satisfaction than doing my job properly and giving a woman her future back.'

'That's exactly what I wanted to hear. Thanks,' I said decisively. 'So let's go ahead on Wednesday… but before we organise it, I have a couple more questions. Let's see… What findings would lead you to recommend chemotherapy?'

'If we find cancerous cells within the lymph nodes.'

'Do you think this cancer has spread to anywhere else?'

'We don't know at this stage, but we will scan you all over, from top to toe, and see if we can find any tumours anywhere else.'

'Right. Okay.' I paused to digest this information so far. 'And what is Tamoxifen?'

'Tamoxifen is a new drug; it was originally a fertility drug but it has the benefits of also blocking the growth of oestrogen-positive tumours. We have been prescribing it for five years now, and it is known currently as a wonder drug.'

'Do I have an oestrogen positive tumour?'

'We don't know at this stage. Once we have removed the tumour we undertake tests on it which take around three weeks for the results to come back.'

'There's a lot we don't know at this stage,' I concluded, more to myself than the surgeon.

'Not without further tests,' he said firmly.

'I understand. It's all quite "wait and see", isn't it? I suppose I'd better settle back into this,' I said.

'I would recommend you do. We can do great things with medicine, but we do need to run tests continuously to make sure we get it right.'

'Do you have any idea what could possibly have triggered it?' I asked, knowing the answer already.

'*That* is the million dollar question,' he snorted. 'If I knew that, then I would not be doing surgery on you next week.

'So nothing outside of what I've read in the literature Liz gave me yesterday?' I persisted. 'Because I don't fit into any of those categories.'

'Sorry. I wish I could tell you, but I can't. I just try to cure you,' he said gently.

'Well, thanks for your time this morning. I won't keep you any longer, and I won't say I'm looking forward to seeing you on Wednesday…' I giggled slightly nervously '… but I'll see you Wednesday.'

'You'll be fine. I'll book you in for Wednesday. And I'll call you back at the beginning of the week to confirm it all. Take care, and don't fret too much in the meantime, thinking up unanswerable questions,' he teased, which finished our conversation on a light, friendly note.

I hung up and sipped my coffee, gazing at my list of questions. The amount of information I was gathering was gaining momentum. This discussion with the surgeon had certainly increased my confidence in him, although I still planned to ask my GP about him as well.

'I'll definitely go with him,' I said, coming into the lounge where Colin was sitting on the sofa, gazing out of the window.

'Why the certainty?' he asked dully.

'Well, because if I go looking for a second opinion without it being on good authority of anyone else, I may end up with the wrong person. It was only to introduce an element of choice, which I can't handle at the moment. I've just spoken to Mr Wintry, and I trust him. He appears a bit arrogant, but I think that's a good thing.'

> *Lesson learned:*
> **Settle back into it. Cancer treatment is a game of Wait and See.**

The rest of Saturday

I sat down, and we both stared silently into the void. The children had moved out to the conservatory, obviously sensing that this was not the time to be hanging around our legs. I briefly wondered whether I should be Talking To Them about what was going on, but I had nothing considered or rehearsed.

'We're supposed to be going out with Chris and Jenny today,' Colin said finally. 'Do you want me to cancel it?'

I didn't answer for a minute. My initial reaction *was* to cancel, but then we would only sit around thinking, thinking, thinking. No, I decided, we should go out with them. I needed the break from all these dreadful scary words that were whirling round my brain, needed to carry on as normal – if not for us, then at least for the children. I laughed hollowly at the word 'normal'. Would my life *ever* be normal again? Everything I understood as normal had just been whisked away from me.

It ended up being the right thing to do, going out with Chris, Jenny and their boys. It distracted all of us; Colin and I even laughed at a couple of jokes. By the end of the day, I was feeling slightly more human again, more ready to stand up and face the imminent onslaught of the coming week. Colin and I spent the evening talking, and I even got a full night's sleep – although I can't say the same for Colin, who I believe stayed up staring wide-eyed at the ceiling all night.

Sunday 20*th* February

The next morning, I got up and took the children to their computer class, and generally tried to instil normality back into a life that has become insane. It was far easier to carry on when you stuck to the humdrum of life. I craved this normality.

I spoke to my mother, my sister and also rang my brothers again, this time getting through to them both. I was getting used to the direction the conversation took as soon as I'd managed to impart my news, trying to manage the other person's feeling of shock and fear. On the whole, most people so far had been very calm and stoical, even managing to make a number of sensible comments and proffer good pieces of advice. I was very impressed – I think I would be a gibbering idiot if a member of my family contacted me with the same news.

By the end of Sunday, Colin was still pale-faced on the sofa. I noticed a collection of plates beginning to gather around him from the various meals I was dishing up: he hadn't touched his food all weekend.

'Will you please eat something?' I begged.

'I'm not hungry,' he muttered, glancing at the toasted cheese sandwiches I'd put before him an hour earlier.

'The last thing we need is for you to get an ulcer, or something,' I said, slightly more sharply than I'd intended. He started eating.

I spent Sunday evening digesting all the information and advice I had been given so far. It was all so much to take in, and the information needed to be churned over frequently, viewing bits from different angles in order to start piecing together the big picture. Currently I felt as though I had only put in ten or fifteen random pieces in a 1,000 piece jigsaw puzzle. There were still so many pieces to fill in.

Further reading "The Shock of Diagnosis"
on the website www.careerkidsandbreastcancer.com

Chapter Three
What causes breast cancer?

Monday 21st February 2000

First day of half-term. Two children at home whilst I tried to arrange the logistics of going to hospital to have a tumour cut out of my breast. Great!

So, first thing Monday morning, I phoned Mr Wintry's secretary to organise some of the private health insurance paperwork and then spoke at length to several people from the office, who had obviously been told by now. The phone rang continuously – I would literally put the phone down from one call when it would ring in my hands. By mid-morning I had talked myself hoarse, and I needed some space. The children had been very good and quiet all morning, glued to the television, and I felt I should do something either with them or for them – or both. After all, this was their half-term holiday!

'Shall we go out?' I asked them, standing in front of the television to get their attention.

They both squirmed in their seats to see past my legs. No. They wanted to watch Power Rangers, Eliot informed me.

'And PowerPuff Girls are on afterwards, and it's my turn to choose next,' said Grace. I shrugged, and went to make myself a coffee. Can't fight good TV.

I sat down at the dining table with a cup of coffee and yesterday's unread newspaper. I flicked through it idly, until an article about exhaustion caught my eye and I settled down to read it.

Almost immediately bells started ringing in my head. It sounded so like me. It was as though the journalist had been a fly on the wall of my life for the last few years before penning the article. I sat back, and tried to pluck out what was for me a classic day – any day from last year would do. I'd get up at seven, have a bath and get dressed before getting the children up. We would all troop downstairs where I would prepare their breakfast, make a cup of coffee for myself, then promptly have to stand over them, nagging them to eat up. Then there was getting dressed time, another session of standing and nagging. Sometimes I would realise that Grace hadn't done her reading homework, so I would have to do that while I half finished getting ready and half looked over Grace's shoulder – oh, and don't forget the preparation of their lunchboxes, which made me laugh at my old longing for having the time to also prepare a salad or a sandwich for myself to take to work. Then there was the usual rush to get three people out of the door – shoes on, hair brushed, coats on, schoolbags, handbags and office bags, find the keys etc etc etc before charging across to the school – which really couldn't be much closer if we'd tried – to drop them off before I leapt into the car and drove round the one-way system to the office. Walking would have been better, and provided some much needed exercise, but it would take five minutes longer and really, every five minutes counted. And anyway, I charged round all day like a maniac – that must constitute exercise. At my calculation, I should have been an eight stone, size ten waif if running around the office shed weight. But it clearly didn't.

Then I would have a frenetic day at work, juggling several different roles, answering eight questions on ten different subjects at a time, and endeavouring to be all things to all people. And indeed, I never remembered to fill my glass at the water fountain despite the fact that I walked, or ran, past it about thirty to fifty times a day. Cups of coffee would appear on my desk from colleagues, and once a week I would make a special effort to do the return round in order to ensure that the magical cups of coffee kept appearing. Lunch was often a packet of crisps from the kitchen if nobody offered to buy me a sandwich when they went up the road, although a large part of the time someone did. Occasionally I would join them for a pub lunch, but even that felt like I was trying to cram in a token bit of social life. I often felt like I returned from a pub lunch with a feeling of 'that's the social bit done, now back to work'.

Charging home from work, eager to see the children but they were often so over-excited and rowdy when I walked in the door, and that made me irritable. Fortunately, my mother-in-law, Rita frequently had them in their pyjamas by the time I got home, and within an hour I would have them in bed. Bedtime story read – frequently a summarised version until Grace learned to read and spotted the yawning gaps of text that I had left out – then lights out and downstairs. In fact, I frequently recall reading to them with my eyelids drooping – or Grace reading her homework books while I slept propped up against the edge of her bed. There's something very lulling about a child reading to you, and I often dropped off to sleep. Grace would wake me with a 'what's that word there?' and I'd try to pretend that I hadn't been kipping.

Once downstairs, I would pour some wine, throw a readymeal in the oven if Colin was going to work till really late, or mix up a quick pasta and throw a jar of sauce over some meat if Colin was going to make it home by ten o'clock. We would then sit in front of the television blankly, absorbing nothing. Rita often attempted conversation, telling me what the children had been up to, but if I wasn't actually asleep on the sofa, or too bombed to react, then I was too distracted with a work issue, and my mind was on anything but the kids. I would often get out some work that I'd brought home and carry on working until eleven or twelve. Colin and I sometimes had brief conversations with each other when either of us had the energy; otherwise we both just craved the silence or the mind-numbingness of television after our demanding days at work. Once in bed, I would fall into a dreamless and exhausted sleep, before the alarm would go off at seven and the whole cycle began again.

What sort of a life is that? I asked myself now.

> *Lesson learned:*
> ***All work and no play makes Jo a sick girl***

The rest of Monday passed in a haze. Neither Grace nor Eliot even bothered to get dressed, but stayed in their pyjamas all day, and I was too bombed to really care. We picked at food and generally slobbed out. When Colin came home, he looked surprised to see that I had already got the children ready for bed – obviously marvelling at how together I was in the face of such adversity.

Normally Colin would just click the TV on and stare at it for half an hour before any conversation began, but tonight he just sat down and the TV screen stayed blank.

'Shall I order pizza?' I suggested, flapping the menu in his direction. He nodded, so I rang up and ordered the usual.

'How was your day?' he asked when I hung up.

'Oh great!' I said in a mock-cheerful voice, picking up my glass of wine and walking over to the sofa. 'I kept walking round the house aimlessly, looking in the cupboards and the fridge for something but never finding it. None of the chairs are right to sit in, I can't find anything I want to eat or drink, the books I'm reading are all wrong, there's nothing interesting to watch on TV... nothing's *right*!'

'Nothing is distracting enough, you mean,' he said.

I sighed as I sat down. Yes, that was it. Colin told me gently that it would take a while to sink in.

'And for it to mean something,' I added.

And so we talked. Colin confessed that he would have been a gibbering wreck by now, incapable of speech, certainly civility. In fact, he said, he'd probably have had to go away for a while, be on his own. As for me, I just wanted to get back to normality, carry on as usual. I didn't think I understood what was going on, what all this meant to me. I was so at-the-beginning of it all, and I didn't know where it's going. Last week my life had been so repetitive and cosy... I could plan ahead, have degrees of certainty and security...

'But all I know for this week is that I go into hospital at 9 am on Wednesday, and they operate at 11 am. A whole week... one plan.'

'Other than to lie in bed and relax, recuperate.' When Colin saw me cringe, he said: 'You're incapable of relaxing, aren't you?'

'If it means lying in bed for days on end, then yes.'

'Have you stopped to wonder why you got this in the beginning?'

'Oh course I have. But no one knows. It's just a lottery,' I said defensively.

'Have you looked at your life over the last five years?'

What? I laughed, recalling my thoughts from earlier that day. Look backwards? Who had time to look backwards, when there was so much coming at you from the front?

'Like what?' Colin demanded.

'Life… things bombard you on a daily basis. Demands from clients, demands from children, demands from the post that comes in through the letterbox every day, the phone ringing with more demands. I mean, this isn't just me, is it? You get this too, don't you?' I looked at Colin.

Of course he did, but there were times when he turned his back on it, and took some time out for himself. 'You never seem to,' he said. 'Ever since I've known you, you seem to be running at ninety miles an hour trying to achieve everything, being all things to all people, and never once stopping to chill, to relax.'

'What's your point?' I said sharply, trying not to feel annoyed at him.

'My point is,' he said soothingly, sensing my rising annoyance, 'take some time for you. Slow down, read some books, watch some videos… stay in bed and relax. Enjoy yourself. This isn't a race to see how quickly you can get better.'

'And what's this got to do with why or how I got this in the beginning?' I argued defensively.

'Jo, people never see themselves as other people see them. Watching you over the years, you've been in some huge race… and no one's body can keep up with that. Eventually the body starts sacrificing parts of its functioning in order to keep pace. You get more stressed as you get more tired, your immune system works harder and harder until at some point it just gives up and says "no more, that's it matey, I've done my bit". You've hit that wall, and now it's payback time. You have to slow down and give your body a chance to recover.' Clearly Colin had done a *lot* of reading on the internet that afternoon.

I felt the tears pouring down my face, and Colin came to comfort me. 'But I want to do both – I want to be a full-time mother to my children as well as have a career and earn an income. I enjoy it.'

'Then do it, but not so manically,' he said. 'I've said it before, and I'll say it again. Let's get in more help. You don't need to exhaust yourself with the housework, and errand-running. We'll get someone else in to do all of that.'

'We can only afford so much home help. And even if I could afford it, you still have to oversee everything. Just getting people in doesn't always get a job done. Half the time you clean up after a cleaner…'

'Don't set yourself such high targets.'

'I don't. In fact, I don't have time to set targets… I just do, do, do all day long.' That was the bit that did my head in most of all, is just the constant *doing*.

I went silent, so Colin pressed home his advantage. Not to *do* anything; just plan. I should try and see how to delegate more to other people. Ask Mum if she could have the children for one weekend in a month so I could have a break; maybe work from home one day a week; get the shopping delivered. I had run myself ragged trying to achieve everything, and, said Colin, 'you do a great job, Jo. The house looks okay, the children are healthy and happy – and I'm sure your filing is all in order. Now sort yourself out. Find something relaxing to do over the next few months while you're recuperating.'

'Like what?'

'Painting, drawing, pottery… I don't know… but something you can potter at. Something that is an end in itself, not a means to an end.'

I was indignant, but Colin insisted that everything was a time and motion study to me – and I knew he was right. I'd spent my life like that: how fast could I do this? How efficiently could I do that? How much could I squeeze into one day? Or one lifetime? It was time to chill. To stop. Do something for the enjoyment of it, not to win any awards or set up a new business.

When the pizza arrived, between mouthfuls we continued talking, with Colin urging me to focus on getting better.

'This might be worse than we think,' I wailed, panic rising up inside. 'I may have secondaries.'

'Well, worrying ain't going to change things. And anyway, you personally can help yourself by taking a positive approach – which you've started doing, and you have to maintain. Don't focus on the spectre of death, because even if this *is* going to kill you, quite frankly it won't be for several years yet. You have a long way to go yet, and that's not taking medical intervention into account.'

'How else?'

'By not worrying about what *might* be. Focus on what *is*. You're scared of the operation – well, focus on that fear and deal with it. Take it one step at a time, and don't fear the chemotherapy until you're having the chemotherapy.'

It sounded great so far, but it was so easy to say, and so difficult to do. After all, this had taken up my every waking thought for twenty-four hours now, and I needed to think of the worst – to address the ghouls and spectres, stare into the face of death, in order to work out what I thought of it.

'But this isn't about death,' insisted Colin. 'This is about an illness, a degenerative illness that may, only *may*, degenerate further and no-one knows at what speed. Contextualise your illness.'

'What do you mean?'

'Put it into context. It's not about an imminent death. It's about the impact of this illness on your life - it's about *how* you're going to *live*.'

My head suddenly cleared. The fog that had been there since Friday afternoon lifted, and I looked at my husband with wide open eyes. He was right! He was so right! It was about the impact, rather than the potential, of the illness. It was the impact on me, on him, on my children, on my work, on my future.

I needed to re-evaluate how I lived my life, and think about what was important in the future, what I wanted for me and for my family. Suddenly I experienced a feeling of hope about the future.

It was as though the possible link between this illness and death had somehow been severed – or at least widened – and I felt I could consider the impact of this illness on my life in a far more practical and positive way.

Lesson learned:
Focus on how to live, not how to die.

Further reading "Exhaustion: The Disease of Today"
on the website www.careerkidsandbreastcancer.com

Chapter Four
Why Me?

Tuesday 22nd February

Plans for today… I was planning to stay calm ahead of my impending hospitalisation the next day. I intended to spend time with the children while getting a bag of stuff together, buying some pyjamas (I didn't have any) and a dressing gown (couldn't possibly take my battered old bathrobe) and slippers (didn't have any). I was also planning to treat myself to some luxury bubble bath and moisturiser – oh, and get some books to read as well.

I lay in bed, enjoying the peace. Colin had left early for work, as he had a lot to get through and needed to get ahead of himself before Wednesday, as he was obviously planning to take the day off. I guessed the children were still asleep. It was only 7.20 am.

I've always loved early mornings – the silence, the newness of the day, the excitement of what good things could happen. An optimist, that's me. A cup half-full. It's funny. I've been so busy over the years that I'd forgotten this was what I used to do as a kid: lie in bed with flutterings of excitement in my tummy as I imagined some of the great things that could happen to me that day.

But as I remembered my past, the present sledge-hammered back into my thoughts. I felt sick. Hospital tomorrow. I've got Breast Cancer, I said to myself. I can't believe this is happening to me. I'm going to have a general anaesthetic tomorrow, and they are going to cut at least a 2cm diameter tumour out of my breast. Arghhghgh!

What conclusion had Colin and I come to last night? That I needed to contextualise my illness, not viewing it as an illness in itself, but thinking of its impact on my life. And this included, firstly, how I was going to get through the treatment; secondly, how I was going to review my approach to my health; and thirdly, how I could safeguard the future, minimise the risks of this illness returning. That and that alone would help me face the future, whatever it should hold. Whatever it should hold, I mused. But still the question loomed: why is this happening to me? Why? Why me?

This nagging thought kept prodding my mind. What did I do? What did I eat? What air did I breathe? What fatal mistake did I make that made my body screw up so badly? Common sense told me that this wasn't something I'd done, but the thought nagged at my mind and I couldn't push it away.

I made myself a coffee and returned upstairs, the morning's paper tucked under my arm. I could hear the children chattering between them, but it sounded like they had started one of their imaginary games. I'd probably have long enough to enjoy my coffee in peace, and read at least some of the paper.

I flicked over the pages until an article about organic food grabbed my attention. I read with growing interest before putting the newspaper down to allow myself time to reflect on it. The article raised some pretty scary facts and statistics about how our food chain was getting totally messed about by the carcinogenic chemicals we spray our crops with. The word 'carcinogenic' leapt off the page at me.

It's weird how, when you are facing some terrible crisis, suddenly every newspaper, TV ad, billboard, whatever, is addressing it. Over the next few months, I was amazed at the frequency of articles directly or indirectly about cancer – particularly about breast cancer. It is such a big issue that it is at the forefront of media the whole time. I'd just never noticed it before.

But this was the first time I had really stopped to read an article about health, environment, organic stuff etc. The long and the short of it was that I'd been eating all the wrong types of food, food fit to give the healthiest person cancer. So, I'd had a hand in my own illness? Or was it the Government's fault for allowing this food to be sold, by not banning all these chemicals, for not legislating against imported, contaminated food and having quality control bodies closely monitoring what the population were eating. After all, cancer treatment blows a huge hole in the NHS budget every year – think how much they could spend on organic farming from the savings made on the NHS!

Further down the article, a phrase caught my eye: 'protecting future generations…' A fact suddenly hit me in the face, one I hadn't acknowledged until now. My diagnosis immediately put my daughter, Grace, into a higher risk category in the future. Reading the facts and figures about chemical residues and carcinogens, I suddenly realised that I *had* to protect my children in a way I'd never previously considered. I had to do my bit to minimise what poisons they consumed. This wasn't just about me.

I could feel myself wading deeper and deeper into the quagmire, into a world that was completely new to me and I had to start learning the basics. Onto the end of my shopping list I added 'Books/magazines re organic lifestyle', just as Grace & Eliot entered the room.

'Can we go downstairs?' Grace asked.

'Okay. I'm getting up now anyway,' I smiled, privately wondering if I seemed the same to them. Or was I different? Did I seem sad? More stressed? Or maybe more patient? Not rushing around? They didn't seem to be looking at me curiously, or oddly. So, I deduced, I must appear the same to them. And that was good. I wouldn't want them worrying.

We had breakfast and got dressed over the course of the next hour, and then I brought out all their jigsaws.

'Let's cover the floor in jigsaws,' I suggested, and they now looked at me curiously, but pleased. We spent a lovely couple of hours doing jigsaws, Grace chattering non-stop, spouting a constant stream of consciousness. Eliot was less wordy, but more expressive as he'd occasionally fling a piece of jigsaw across the room because 'it wouldn't work'. I would patiently help him with his frustration, fetching the misbehaving piece of jigsaw and subtly pointing out where it should go. By lunchtime, I was subconsciously looking at my watch as I was planning to go into Kingston after lunch to shop.

Unfortunately, kids being kids decided to play up that afternoon. Eliot, who had just turned four, didn't want to be strapped into a buggy and pushed around Bentalls' nightie department. He wanted to run around, scream, to be a power-ranger or a buffalo. It was a nightmare, and for the first time in my life I completely and utterly lost my temper at the both of them. Having spent a frustrating half-hour alternating my attention between choosing a nightdress, dressing gown and slippers, and hissing at Grace and Eliot to stop running between the racks of the clothes, I departed to the sound of a loud, collective sigh of relief from the shop staff.

I tried bribing the kids, with the promise of sweeties, to be good while I endeavoured to choose a couple of books at Waterstones. But I like to spend at least an hour browsing the shelves to carefully choose my reading material; instead I had to choose and run because their behaviour was getting out of control. I could feel my temper rising. They whinged the whole way back to the car, and as I unlocked the car doors, something inside me snapped. I started screaming at them, then thumping the car with my balled up fists – aware of a couple of women across the car park by the ticket machine staring at me. I put my head on my folded arms, leaning against the car, and cried from the depths. The rational part of me was kind of glad, as I hadn't allowed myself to let go until now, and I'd felt like I was ready to burst inside. Quashing all that misery cannot be good.

Finally I raised my head off my arms and looked at the children. Eliot was crying, still strapped into his buggy, and Grace was big-eyed, staring at me and clutching onto the side of the buggy.

'I'm sorry. I shouldn't have shouted at you two,' I said gently, wiping my eyes. The women across the car park watched, probably to see if I was going to thump the kids or something, I supposed. I ignored them, and squatted down beside the buggy, gathering both children into my arms. 'You've not done anything that bad – I was just upset about something else. I'm having a bad few days, and there's something I'm unhappy about. But I shouldn't have shouted at you. It's not your fault.'

Eliot carried on crying; Grace stroked my arm. After a short while, I stood up and started to calmly load them into the car. 'Let's go home,' I said, deciding to abandon the rest of my shopping trip.

Mum was there when I got back. She'd let herself in with her key, and was in the kitchen making coffee when we walked in the door. She said something about good timing, and she'd make me one as well. Then she stopped abruptly when she saw my face. I always look like such a road accident after I've been crying – puffy, white face, red eyes... it's not pretty.

I saw her eyes go instinctively to the children to see if they were also in a state of high emotion, and she registered Eliot's blotchy face and Grace's big-eyed, pale look.

'Bad day?' Mum said. I started to crumple again, and buried my face in a pile of tissues. Mum led me to a chair and suggested to the children that she put a video on for them.

She placed a steaming mug of coffee down in front of me, and waited till I was able to form words and explain what had happened.

'It's really not about today,' I added. 'I think I was just reacting to the diagnosis – finally. And fear of tomorrow. Fear of the general anaesthetic. Fear of what they'll find. Fear that they'll cut my breast off while I'm out for the count, and that I won't have a say in it. Fear that he's a shite surgeon, that I've picked the wrong guy. But it wasn't fair on the kids. I shouldn't have scared them like that.'

'They'll survive it, Jo. It's not such a bad thing that they're a part of what's happening – you're all one family, and what affects you also affects them. It's probably better that they see you crying, that they feel part of what they can probably sense anyway.'

I shook my head, although I knew there was a lot of sense in her words. 'They still didn't need to see me lose it.'

'They'll be fine.' Mum stroked my hair momentarily. I was trying to stop crying, but part of me just wanted to curl up into a ball and carry on. I think Mum sensed this.

'Would you prefer that I took the children now, and give you some time alone?' she suggested. I paused, then nodded. I hadn't packed any bags for them, but Mum made short work of throwing some clothes etc together and within fifteen minutes the children were installed in her car, waving goodbye to me – Eliot's face beginning to crumble in tears, and Grace bearing an uncertain smile... or was it a reassuring smile?

Further reading "Surviving Stress; surviving ill-health"
on the website www.careerkidsandbreastcancer.com

Chapter Five
Why not me?

Tuesday 22nd February 2000 – early evening
The house was silent and empty. I could cry my heart out now, and get all the misery out of me. But the moment had passed. I didn't feel like it now. Instead I started clearing the house up, putting away jigsaws and toys, moving from room to room to put everything back where it belonged. As I ambled around, I was deep in thought, sorting out all my thoughts, ordering and filing. I could feel my head clearing a bit.

After an hour, the house looked neat and tidy again. I rewarded myself with a cup of coffee, and pulled out some of the organic magazines I had bought on the hoof in the bookshop. I settled into an armchair and became completely immersed in the articles, exploring deeper the cocktail of carcinogenic chemicals that we call a 'foodchain' – my whole diet and lifestyle of high fat, high sugar, low activity was a modern phenomenon called slow death. We are all living ourselves to death.

> *Lesson learned:*
> ***The question shouldn't be WHY ME but rather WHY NOT ME?***

I decided to do a little experiment, and check through my fridge and cupboards to see what was in the foods I was eating. It was scary. Chemicals, e-numbers, organophosphates, saturated fats – it was all there. There was very little natural content in any of my collection of tins, jar sauces and ready meals.

Never one to do things by halves, I decided that I might as well go food shopping and see what organic food was on the shelves, particularly as I realised that our fridge and food cupboard were running very low on supplies. I hadn't been shopping in a week, and I couldn't go into hospital and leave Colin with an old lump of cheese and wrinkling mushrooms.

An hour later, I returned from my shopping expedition loaded up with organic fruit and vegetables, organic butter, milk, yoghurt, cereals, mustard, chicken and lamb, eggs and some jar sauces. Colin was already home and wondering where I was. As I unpacked, I told him the shocking facts about carcinogens in intensively farmed food.

'There are around 80,000 chemicals in circulation today, most of which end up on our food and can leave carcinogenic residues on what we eat. From now on, we're going organic – we're going to eat good and wholesome stuff, free of chemicals, additives, preservatives and stuff fit to give you cancer.'

Colin listened and nodded, seemingly unconvinced, but wisely elected to let me carry on rolling.

'The supermarkets are beginning to store a fair amount of organic stuff, but according to the article in the paper, there are also some organic box schemes which deliver. I'll have to find out about it,' I continued.

'I think this is very laudable, but let's not go overboard,' said Colin, dipping his hand into the chocolate Minibix packet and crunching away.

'Overboard? Do you realise that this isn't just about me – although a large part of it is. I want to do my level best to avoid *this* coming back again, but it's also about Grace and Eliot. I have to stop feeding them chemical residues right here and now in order to protect their bodies – and to support the organic movement in protecting the land that they need in the future for them, and for their children, and *their* children – all *our* descendents!' I said passionately.

'When you get a bee in your bonnet…' Colin said mildly, picking up the newspaper and deciding to have a read of it himself. I busied myself with preparing some organic chicken, topped by an organic sauce and accompanied by an organic side salad.

'There. Now we can taste the difference.' I put them down and then disappeared to get the fruit juice.

Colin tasted his meal. To him it tasted exactly the same, and he said so.

'Nonsense! This lettuce definitely tastes, well, *greener* – and the carrot is so *orange*-tasting!' I enthused.

'I think you're imagining it,' Colin said.

'Not at all. You can virtually taste the earth. This, my dear man, is going to be the stuff that prevents your children getting this disease when they're older.' I shovelled the food into my mouth, as though each mouthful of natural, organic goodness was shrinking the tumour. Colin looked at me doubtfully, but said nothing. He turned the page of the magazine and read the next article about the dangers of milk *(website article "Breast Cancer dangers in milk")*.

'So you think this is all due to dairy food, do you?' Colin said, putting down the magazine and finishing his meal.

I nodded. 'And I read that in the UK, one in twelve women is diagnosed with breast cancer, and they think the figure is higher in the south of England – could even be one in six women there. Women in the States have a one in eight chance, and women in the Far East have a one in ten thousand chance. Hullo! Can I go to the Far East then, please?'

'By why such an incredibly different statistic?'

'Precisely. That's what the article was about. Diet.'

Apparently, an Oriental woman, living on an Oriental diet, massively reduces her chances of developing cancer, whereas an Oriental woman living in the West on a Western diet will, within one or two generations, develop the same risk factor as other Western women. And the fundamental difference lies in diet. Orientals don't eat dairy produce, for example, whereas we eat it by the gallon. And what I couldn't understand was that Governmental Health bodies were trying to get children and women to have even *more* dairy, not less.

'Obviously osteoporosis is more of a threat in terms of numbers than cancer is.' Colin shrugged.

'Not quite as life-threatening though.'

'I think I'd trust the Government before some unknown quack with a theory.'

'Why? The Government used to recommend bread and dripping for dinner – now the dripping causes cholesterol. And you had to have an egg a day, now they cause listeria. They backtrack on all health warnings.'

'This isn't the Government changing their minds. This is an unknown quack expounding a viewpoint. It doesn't make her right,' Colin argued.

But I was adamant. 'Every theory has a thesis, an antithesis, then a synthesis. Jane Plant is challenging our current beliefs with a new thesis, and society needs radical thinkers who challenged popular beliefs; this in turn leads to a synthesised and moderated agreement once conformists and radicals have battled it out with each other.' I argued.

'This isn't a time for you to go radical.' he countered.

He was happy to go organic, but he didn't agree with cutting out dairy. 'If you cut dairy out of your diet, you'll get osteoporosis. It just leads to other problems.'

'If you eat enough greens, you'll get loads of calcium,' I argued based on my new-found knowledge.

'How many's enough? A field of greens a day? Better make sure they're organic.' Colin laughed.

I laughed back, not bothering to answer. Colin loved being provocative in arguments. I'd already made up my mind to consider cutting out dairy, though not without speaking to a nutritionist first, and finding out what I had to replace it with.

Colin urged me to do it sensibly. 'I don't want you going all alternative on me, and thinking that diet alone can get rid of cancer. You need conventional medicine like chemo and radio therapy—'

'Of course!' I interrupted quickly. 'I wouldn't consider not having those treatments. Believe you me, I want to take out the biggest insurance policy going here to minimise the risk of this cancer ever returning. If it means considering changing my diet *alongside* conventional treatments, then I'll do it. But one won't replace the other.'

Colin nodded, and I could see he was trying to frame his next sentence carefully. I waited, fiddling with the stem of my wine glass as though preoccupied, in order to give him time. Finally he spoke. 'I want you to know that I'm behind you, beside you, whatever, all the way. Investigate all these things, and do everything you can to minimise your risk factor. But don't be irrational, okay? Please don't go off on wild goose chases, expending all your time, money, energy and faith on coffee enemas and so-called cancer-curing vitamins from the small ads. And don't shut me out,' he begged.

'I promise,' I said sincerely. 'We're in this together.'

We sat down later to watch a film to distract our minds from the next day. Both of us were nervous. We'd talked ourselves hoarse in the last four days, and now we just craved peace. Colin let me choose the film *and* hold the remote. Little demonstrations of love and concern!

I tried to concentrate on the film but it hadn't caught my attention and my mind kept wandering – I think I'd have been hard-pushed to have found a film that would have held my attention that evening. Instead I sat there, looking at cancer from every angle possible, trying to understand what point it served in my life. These questions kept hammering at my mind, giving me no peace. The more I thought about it, the crosser I found myself getting. If cancer was caused by chemicals, then I – as well as everyone else – had a right to know what I was consuming. I needed to investigate the whole food issue really closely, to truly understand what I ate every day, and to make sure the dangerous foods were eliminated not only from my diet, but also Grace and Eliot's.

By the time I went to bed, I had worked myself up into a real stew and had decided that my mission was to find out the truth about food, then to shout it from the rooftops to stop such awful farming practices.

> *Lesson learned:*
> **Modern day farming practices may contribute to the increase in cancer**

That night, I had a nightmare. I was being led down a long, dark corridor, but I couldn't see the shadowy person who was holding my arm although I could feel the pressure of his hand around my upper arm. He was talking in a low, quiet voice, telling me reassuringly, 'We'll just give you a little injection and you'll go to sleep for a little while. When you wake up it will all be over.' The voice was hushed and reassuring, but I heard menace and fought an urge to run. The corridor was so long, so quiet, so dark. The closed doors, spaced at regular intervals along the corridor, were also menacing, and the bright light at the end of the corridor scared me. I knew it was the operating theatre, and I could see the over-exposed doctors moving around an empty operating table. I suddenly realised that if I went in, I would never come back out. This was death and I wasn't ready yet. Not for years yet. I tried to turn and run, but the hand clamped down tightly on my arm. I screamed.

I sat up in bed, shaking and sweating, and switched the light on. Colin wasn't there – no doubt he was sleeping on the sofa downstairs as I was sleeping so restlessly at the moment, and disturbing him. I wondered if I'd screamed out loud, but the lack of response from Colin told me that I hadn't. There was silence, apart from the pounding of my heart in my ribcage. I decided to get out of bed. After all, there was no way I could just lie down and go back to sleep.

I padded into Grace and Eliot's room, and my heart skipped a beat at their empty beds. Then I remembered they were at my mother's house. Instead I went back to bed and conjured up their lovely little faces. They were the most precious things in my life, and I knew beyond doubt that if ever their lives or safety were threatened, I would fight to the death to save them.

How then could I fight to save myself, in order to be with them? The thought of one of them dying before me was crucifying, but the thought of me not being there for them was just as overwhelming. I had to be there for them. I had to live. There was no alternative. No choice. Even though you don't get a say in that matter. And what made me different from any other loving mother,

other loving mothers who had died? Nothing. Absolutely sodding nothing.

Despite this, I vowed that I had to give myself the best sporting chance, and I resolved to do anything, however far-fetched and tenuous it might be - it could improve my chances of fighting this disease off.

Further reading "Organic debates"
on the website www.careerkidsandbreastcancer.com

Chapter Six
Surviving hospital

February 23rd 2000 – 11.30am

My operation was scheduled for 11.30 Wednesday morning, and I had been told to arrive at the hospital around 9-9.30. By 9.15 I was checked in, shown to my room and unpacked. The room was very pleasant with an en suite bathroom. Ah! The luxuries of private health – although I had read that you were actually better off in an NHS hospital nowadays, because they have the full infrastructure and requirements if you need any emergency treatment such as post-operative resuscitation. But I wasn't going to allow that to put me off.

The butterflies in my stomach were making me feel quite queasy now, and I desperately tried to stop thinking about anaesthetics and scalpels by reading a magazine my sister Kate had sent to me, which had an interesting article about Surviving Hospital. To gain some sense of control over my situation, I had dutifully carried out some of its recommendations so I was well prepared with books, TV guides, chocolates, magazines and a small amount of money, as well as having rung my family and given them my phone number.

Colin hovered around the room, trying to look calm but I could sense his nervousness and misery. A succession of medical people came in, wrote down details, asked questions, took my temperature and blood pressure, and generally made small talk. Finally Mr Wintry came in.

'Hello, Joanna. And how are you today?' he said cheerily.

'Fine, just fine.' I said untruthfully. I was a bag of nerves. 'I feel a bit sick,' I added.

'Well, you're in the right place,' he joked. I smiled weakly. Though the procedure had been previously explained to me, he proceeded to describe in detail (though thankfully not too graphic) what he was going to do. When he had finished, he asked if I had any further questions.

'What are the chances of you not getting all the cancerous The nurse came out of the bathroom to help me up onto the trolley that would take me to theatre, and she kindly held the back of my gown closed to maintain some sense of decency in front of the porter.

'Wouldn't you rather walk down there?' Colin asked. I shook my head. My legs were rapidly turning to jelly, and I suspected that I would either collapse or make a last minute dash for the door.

'Now, we're just going to go for a little joy-ride,' said the porter, as though I was five, not thirty-five. I let it go and just nodded politely. We swung out into the corridor and started whizzing along. I passed some pedestrians on the way, and felt such a fraud for being wide-awake yet pushed along on a bed. We went left round one corner, down another corridor, right, then left and suddenly we were in a bright room – the preparation room outside the operating theatre. Nurses and anaesthetists milled around busily. We paused at the door, and Colin bent over and kissed me. Neither of us could say anything, and I think each was fighting back the tears so as not to alarm the other. He stepped back and I heard him giving his phone number to the nurse, with instructions to be called as soon as I was out of theatre. The doors flapped shut.

A Scandinavian-looking and sounding nurse hove into view, wearing a cheery smile. 'Hello, I'm Birgit. I'm the anaesthetist. How are you feeling?'

I burst into tears.

'There is nothing to be scared of. I'm going to put a little butterfly in the back of your hand and very soon you will be asleep.'

The tension finally got too much, and I couldn't stop myself. 'That's what I'm scared of – you sending me to sleep,' I muttered between sobs.

Birgit bent her knees slightly to be more at my level. 'You will be fine. The next thing you know you will be sitting up in bed telling me how easy it all was.'

'And telling us all about her children,' added another nurse to Birgit. 'Joanna's got two children – Grace and Eliot.'

'Oh, I love the name Grace,' Birgit said.

'What made you pick that name?' asked the nurse on the other side of me. I knew it was a ruse to get me to look away from Birgit as she inserted the canula, and to distract me as the anaesthetic took effect. Again, I let it ride and decided to play along, desperate to feel calm again. I'd always heard that if you were stressed when you were put to sleep you would wake up stressed and crying. I took a couple of deep breaths.

'We'd chosen the name by the time I was three months pregnant,' I began, feeling the edges of my vision going blurry and my limbs going heavy. I pressed on, the child in me setting a challenge to see how much I could say before I went to sleep. 'I had a great aunt called Grace and…we…always… ' I slurred, then darkness descended.

'Hello, you're back in your room now, and it's all over,' said a woman's voice. I fought through the darkness and heaviness, and tried to say something. I heard my voice, and then darkness descended again.

'I'm just taking your obs,' a voice said, and I felt my right arm being moved around. I nodded in acquiescence and carried on sleeping.

'I'm just doing your obs again,' a voice came at my side again. 'Are you feeling alright?'

'Yes,' I managed to mutter, allowing the sleepiness to claim me again.

'Hello, I'm just going to take your blood pressure and temperature,' said a voice coming into the room. I peered through my heavy eyelids and saw a nurse coming round to my right side.

'What time is it?'

'Twenty past four,' came the reply. I nodded and went back to sleep.

'I'm just going to do your obs,' said a nurse coming into the room.

'Again?' I muttered, waking up suddenly.

'Yes, we have to keep checking you to make sure you're stable,' she smiled, popping the thermometer in my mouth.

'What time is it?' I mumbled through nearly-closed, dry lips.

'Nearly six.' The nurse deftly wrapped the blood pressure cloth around my arm and started pumping. I was aware of the blood pounding round my brain. I lay quietly, half watching the nurse and half sliding back into sleep again.

'Hello, how are you feeling?' said a nurse coming into the room.

'Let me guess… my obs?' I said weakly, opening my eyes.

'Cor-rect,' she smiled. I lay silently as the nurse got on with it. I still felt incredibly sleepy.

I woke to see a nurse holding a tray of food and asking if I wanted anything to eat or drink. All I wanted was a gallon of water; my throat was parched. I tried to sit up, and my head pounded. The nurse helped me, and I managed a sip of water before lying back down thankfully.

'Your husband left only half an hour ago. He said he'd be back by eight thirty in the morning – or before if you need him,' said the nurse. I nodded, and drifted off to sleep again. They must have pumped some powerful sleep-inducing pain-relief into me, as I then slept through the rest of the night.

Thursday 24*th* February, 6am

I woke early the next morning, my head still pounding but curiously little pain in my breast. Somebody had changed me into my new nightdress, and I propped myself up to have a look at my surgery. There was nothing to see but dark-flesh coloured bandages – curiously flat. *Did they remove the whole breast?* I wondered dimly, still fairly numb from the anaesthetic.

'How's my patient this morning?' said a cheery voice from the door. Mr Wintry was doing his early morning rounds. He made some small talk as he inspected the bandaging around my breast and under my arm, and it was at that point I discovered I had a tube coming out of the side of me, draining a bloody-looking fluid. I gagged momentarily.

'We also removed the lymph nodes while you were out,' he began. I wondered at his terminology, picturing them operating on my arm while the rest of me was out shopping; then wondered at my own lack of emotion. Mr Wintry looked serious, so I composed my face ready for the next onslaught of bad news.

He had tested the tumour to confirm its malignancy, and even at this very late stage of the day I hoped for him to say that he was wrong; that it had been a benign lump. But it was indeed malignant. And because the first place cancerous cells invariably travel to is the lymph nodes under the arm, he had taken out all the lymph nodes he could. 'We got fifteen,' he told me, 'so I'm pretty satisfied that we got them all.'

I nodded, and muttered something like 'oh, that's good' like it was a football score. 'Is my breast still there?' I asked after a moment.

Mr Wintry looked surprised, then nodded, understanding my question. 'Oh yes. That's a high-pressure dressing to minimise the risk of any fluid build-up in the cavity – which is why you also have that drain.'

I nodded again, and plumped back onto the pillows, exhausted.

Mr Wintry said he'd come back in to see how I was doing tomorrow. I'd probably be here for around three to five days. In the meantime, I was to rest and not worry. 'The cancer, to all intents and purposes, is out now,' he assured me. 'We will be running tests on the tumour to see whether it's hormone reaction, and see how many of the lymph nodes were infected.' Mr Wintry looked at me long and hard before concluding, 'You'll be fine.'

It was the first positive statement I'd heard from him. But I was shattered, so I turned over gently (so as not to disturb the tubes sticking out of me) and went to sleep.

> *Lesson learned:*
> **After the operation, you no longer have cancer**

Thursday 24th February, 10am

Colin was there when I woke up a couple of hours later. I still felt very muzzy and unable to say much. 'You look well,' he joked, shocked at how awful his wife looked. He'd also got a real fright when he walked into the room the evening before. When they'd brought me back from the operating room someone had changed me into my own pyjamas, which fitted quite closely, and at first he thought they'd removed my left breast. He'd shot back out of the room and collared a passing nurse who explained the principles of high pressure dressings which had pretty much flattened the breast. It was still there, she reassured him.

I smiled at his joke. 'I'm a bit dull at the moment,' I muttered through numb lips.

'Well, I'll go then. I was expecting wine and sparkling wit,' he said. 'How does it feel?'

'Numb. I can't feel it at all.'

'And you? How do you feel?'

'Faint, dizzy, cotton-woolly, pounding head – the usual post-operative stuff,' I shrugged and told him about Mr Wintry's dawn visit. 'And I have a lovely pot of gloop being drained out of me.' I pointed down to the other side of my bed. Colin remained seated, not caring to see what was being drained out.

My mum had called, and my sister, and both my brothers – as well as Colin's mum. He had told them all that the op went well... as well as we'd been told so far, anyway. Colin sat down heavily on the chair, rubbing his hands momentarily into his face. He looked shattered.

'How's work?' I asked, moving the conversation away from me.

'I don't know. I'm just turning up to the office at the moment, but I don't think I'm being very effective.'

We talked a bit more, then went silent. Neither of us really had the energy to talk and I was beginning to feel particularly sleepy again, despite it only being nine o'clock. The hospital day always starts so ridiculously early. Colin picked up the TV remote and put his feet up. I dozed off.

Every half hour or so, I opened my eyes and smiled at him. He patted my hand, gave me some water and made some idle chat. It must have been mid-morning when I opened my eyes briefly and saw Colin sitting uncomfortably in the upright chair, flicking through daytime TV for something to watch. I told him to come back later that evening, as I just wanted to sleep and it seemed pointless for him to sit there watching me. I wasn't awake long enough to see whether he was relieved.

24th-25th February 2000

The hours passed quite quickly in those calm, peaceful surroundings. The flowers started coming in, and the cards, as word slowly spread around the wider family and friends. Colin came in to see me morning and evening, and I had my own telephone beside my bed so I could call my family. I attempted to watch TV, but even in my numbed state I found it too tedious. I felt groggy from the anaesthetic, and this was exacerbated by the stiflingly warm atmosphere common to hospitals. I was urged to walk around to help eliminate the effects of the anaesthetic, and I drank loads of water to flush my system out. The nurses told me the frequent walks would help to minimise the possibility of getting a thrombosis, so I complied obediently.

Lesson learned:
Follow all medical advice – drink lots and walk plenty; do your exercises.

On one of my many walks I found a reading room with loads of old newspapers and magazines, and that is where I ended up spending most of my time between my brief jaunts. I leafed through them all, hungrily looking for something of interest to read and found loads of articles about cancer research studies, nutrition etc. I couldn't believe the copious amount of articles about cancer, the links between cancer and diet, about diet generally, the state of the nation's food chain, what genetic modification was. It was fascinating.

The more I read, the more my fears and my resolve grew. Standard intensive farming methods were bad enough; now, reading about genetic modification, my fears deepened. And not just for me, but for my children. Data was steadily being amassed about the chemicals in our food and intensive farming methods.

Who could possibly tell at this stage the long-term effects of consuming genetically modified products? There were no long-term studies, and it wasn't right for scientists to promote GM foods yet.

As far as I was concerned, it actually made very sound sense that, given the complexity of the human body and its digestive processes, if you alter the structure of the food you consume, you must at some point affect how the human body processes this food. It could set off different genetic modifications within the body, and these would be impossible to predict at this stage. My resolve to use only organic and non-genetically modified food grew stronger.

Many other debates raged on in the newspapers. Did dairy food cause breast cancer? What of sodium laurel sulphate in hair products? And triclosan in toothpaste? Everything seemed to cause cancer. Now my head was really spinning, and I was genuinely puzzled. Should I drink milk and eat cheese? Or should I not? The counter-arguments to Professor Jane Plant's theories were strongly put but in fact shallow, all of them expressing outrage but none actually going as far as to disprove Plant's theories. But who to believe? Where was the truth amongst all the theories and counter theories?

I wondered why all the experts couldn't just be put together in one room to thrash it out once and for all. At least the arguments going backwards and forwards over the chemical residues were directly attacking each other's point of view, and not being at all woolly about it. Despite a good counter-argument put up by the 'there are no residues' brigade, I still supported the 'oh yes there are residues' camp.

I was also dejected when I read how all the personal products were filled with chemicals, some of which could be carcinogenic. Having just spent a fortune clearing out and replacing my food stores, it looked like I would have to clear out all the shelves in my bedroom and bathroom and replace all the personal products. Shampoo and conditioners, anti-perspirants, skin creams, sun creams… the list was endless. By the time I had put down the last magazine I was no longer asking why *I* had got cancer, but rather why hadn't *everyone* got cancer? Certainly if there was any truth in this information, everyone was heading for cancer – and wasn't that what The Ecologist was saying? It was truly scary.

When I got tired of reading, I would phone friends to tell them what was happening. Now that the operation had been done and I no longer had breast cancer (as far as we knew), I started to find it easier to tell people. I realised how subconsciously a lot of the stress had also been bound up in my fear of anaesthetics, and now that was out of the way, I could concentrate on recuperation and treatment. With each phone call, I got used to dodging the answer to the first 'How are you', and chatted for a bit before coming out with my news. The shock was palpable each time, expressed more often than not in a gasp before the other person managed to gather their wits to talk.

Between phone calls, I would walk and read some more. The nurses couldn't believe how contained and absorbed I was. They never heard a peep out of me. I was either sleeping, reading or on the phone. Mr Wintry called me his star patient.

On Friday, he came in to see me with a smile on his face. 'I'm very impressed with how you've dealt with the whole operation. Your positive attitude has really contributed to a speedy recovery from the op itself.'

'Thank you,' I said, pleased, as Mr Wintry had struck me as someone who was very difficult to please.

'So you can go home today.'

'Oh great!' I said enthusiastically. I was longing to see my babies, to sit in my own environment and watch some decent films. 'I'll phone Colin and tell him. But he probably won't be able to fetch me until late this afternoon…'

'That's fine. No rush.' Mr Wintry checked me over and signed me out, so I was free to leave when I wanted. 'Liz, the breast care counsellor, will be round to show you some exercises to care for your arm and stop it seizing up. Do them religiously, as it makes a huge difference,' he advised.

'And the results from the other tests?'

'It may be the end of today, or it may be Monday. I'll chase them up.' And he was gone.

Liz came round to my room mid-morning and we had a chat. She showed me how to do the post-operative exercises, and gave me a printed poster of the exercises which I vowed to put up on the wall to encourage me to do the exercises. I had, by chance, brought a front opening maternity bra with me. This turned out to be really beneficial as I had limited movement in my left arm. The removal of the lymph nodes requires moving (and therefore bruising) muscles and nerves out of the way. Sometimes the nerves remain dead forever. Which would be great for future underarm waxing, but you are advised against doing this.

Friday 25th February, 6pm

I was sitting in the chair beside the hospital bed, waiting for Colin and watching some rubbish on TV when the phone rang later that same day. 'Hello?'

'Hi, it's Mr Wintry,' said a voice at the other end. 'How are you feeling? I was hoping to have contacted you before you left the hospital, as the results from the tests came through last night, by which time I had left. I've just come in to the office now and seen them.'

'Oh.' My hand tightened on the telephone. *Please, please, please let them be negative.*

'I'm afraid there are one or two lymph nodes affected, which is still very early.'

'But what does that mean?' I asked, my brain deserting me as once again I resorted to short, simple questions.

'It means that the cancer had already travelled to your lymph nodes under your arm. We call it a stage two node positive tumour – which is still in the early stages of cancer. More than four lymph nodes indicates a more advanced breast cancer. We got fifteen lymph nodes out, which is good. So I'm confident we have got everything.'

'And what next?'

'First, we allow you to recuperate from this surgery, then we will commence a programme of treatment which is likely now to include chemotherapy and radiotherapy.'

My heart plummeted, and I felt sick. 'Okay,' I said, my eyes watering.

'Come to see me next week, and we will take off the dressing from your breast, and the stitches from under your arm. We can then talk about timing.'

'Okay.'

'And don't worry. Chemotherapy isn't all that bad. This is the new millennium, and we can minimise all the side-effects.'

I asked Mr Wintry what the chances were of this having gone anywhere else, and he admitted there was a chance, although it was small, because they had caught it at two lymph nodes, not four. But they would scan me from top to toe to check.

We said goodbye, and I hung up as Colin walked in the door. I looked at him and started crying. 'I'm not getting off at Junction 2, but going up to Junction 3,' I wept. Colin understood immediately, and held me.

'Apparently chemo isn't so bad,' he tried to comfort me.

I sniffed. 'It doesn't make any odds either way. I'm having it regardless, even if it's the most unpleasant treatment in the world. After all, it's a known cure, and that, when all's said and done, is what I want.'

He asked me how many I had to have; I didn't know. There was so much I didn't know, but all would be revealed as we went along. I had to see the oncologist in a couple of weeks, and he would plan out my treatment.

'In any case, he said even if it hadn't gone up to the lymph nodes, he possibly would have recommended chemotherapy anyway, just to be on the safe side. They intend to get another thirty-five years at least out of me.' I forced a smile through my tears.

Colin felt sick. The thought of them pumping toxic chemicals into his wife made his stomach churn. 'Do you have to have chemo?'

'It maximises my chances of survival.'

He nodded. 'You'll probably outlive me.'

'Is that supposed to be reassurance?' I snapped, as Colin stood up and picked up my bags.

Friday 25th February, 8pm

Back home, I was feeling shattered and decided to go upstairs to bed. But despite my exhaustion, sleep evaded me for many hours and I lay in bed, staring wide-eyed into the darkness wondering where this 'cancer journey' was taking me. I was still awake when Colin came into the bedroom at around midnight. We looked at each other, words not required, and Colin sat down heavily on the edge of the bed, his shoulders slumped and his eyes haunted.

'What happened to all these choices they talked about in the beginning? There don't seem to be any choices at all – none that we're able to make at any rate,' he said finally.

'Not if I want to live, no,' I agreed, and we remained for a long time in silence until Colin finally went back downstairs, unable to sleep.

> *Lesson learned:*
> **Settle back into it – cancer treatment is like a motorway made up of many junctions**

Further reading "Surviving hospital"
on the website www.careerkidsandbreastcancer.com

Chapter Seven
Back to normal?

26th February – 9th March 2000

Life began to resume *something* resembling normality over the next few weeks, insofar as Colin went to work each day, the children were back at school from their half-term break, and Rita was back looking after the children. The only abnormal thing was that I was sitting around at home rather than charging around at work. I found this inactivity incredibly frustrating. Even if I had felt capable, Colin and Rita were watching over me like hawks to make sure I didn't suddenly start putting up some shelves or surreptitiously painting a room. So I started writing a diary...

I had a constant dull ache on my left side and the stitches felt really tight, as though they were stitched to the side of my head and pushing my shoulder up. One day I caught sight of myself in the mirror and realised I was walking around with my left shoulder hiked up higher than my right – I subsequently kept reminding myself to drop my left shoulder. But I was absolutely religious about doing my exercises, and quickly found my arm loosening up day by day.

Saturday 26th February

Saturday 26th February was my sister's birthday. I don't know now if I rang her and wished her happy birthday as I was still living in the post-operative cotton-wool world. But this date never goes past without me at least thinking of you.

Sunday 27th February

My younger brother Ian was over from Hong Kong on a flying visit, and came over to Kingston on the Sunday – two days after I had come out of hospital. It's odd, but when I was sitting around doing nothing, I felt so normal and well. The moment a social occasion arose, even the exertion of chatting just drained me. So

Colin and Ian did most of the chatting, and I sat back and listened – despite the fact that I wanted to chatter, as Ian's visits are irregular and I miss both my brothers. We're a close family, and we'd always seen a lot of each other when they both lived in London.

We walked very slowly into Kingston to get some lunch, and went shopping for CDs and films. Having spent most of the week in hospital, I was craving an outing and reluctant to admit that I felt really rather weak by the time we had walked the short distance to town. By the time we got home, Ian had to leave to catch his plane back to Hong Kong, and I retired to bed. A short and sweet visit, and we always manage to just pick up from where we left off from a previous visit.

Monday 28th February

My next visitor, on the Monday evening, was Pete, the managing director from my office. He said I looked fine, but I felt extremely grey. We chatted for a while, him trying to reassure me about all the positive 'cancer' stories, the great treatments available etc. I wasn't up for long conversations and I'd been subconsciously worrying about what would happen vis-à-vis work and salary. Pete reassured me that the company would continue to pay my salary throughout my treatment, which was a huge weight off my mind. Financially, we'd have been in the proverbial poo if I stopped earning, as Colin had only just set up his own business nine months earlier. The stress that would accompany a lack of salary would certainly not aid my treatment. I promised Pete I would advise them as soon as I knew a return-to-work date. In my naiveté I had drawn a line through three weeks from the middle of February to the second week in March. At that point I really thought I would be back at work within the month! It was to be eight months before I returned to work.

I asked about how my workload was being handled, but Pete had only just got back into the office after a week's holiday, only to be told about my sudden departure, so he was still rather shocked. I told him that I was more than happy to take phone calls and answer any questions people had on my projects. Pete shrugged it all off and reiterated that I should just concentrate on looking after myself.

29ᵗʰ February – 9ᵗʰ March 2000

Flowers, cards and letters arrived daily, and the phone did not stop ringing – Rita could not believe how often it rang. The house had been virtually silent during the day for years, with only the radio quietly playing music and chatting to itself in the background. Suddenly every fifteen minutes was punctuated by the shrill call of the phone. She had started off by answering it, but noticed that I was finding it very difficult to spend *all* day talking about breast cancer. In the end, Rita and I agreed it was better to let the answer-phone take the call. I found that after repeating my story several times, I was tired. I was tired of talking, tired of talking about myself, and tired of hearing my own story. Which was good, I told myself. I had accepted reality to the point of boredom. In the end, I changed the message on my answer-phone, giving my e-mail address so that well-wishers could e-mail me – then I could call people back when I had the energy.

> ### Lesson learned:
> ## Let the answer phone take the calls; return the calls when you feel up to it.

Along with the cards, family and friends were also sending my newspaper clippings as they knew my love of information and feeling in control. I read these articles assiduously; so many were very timely.

Below are excerpts from two that particularly inspired me:

The Lavender Trust – A legacy

During their course of treatment for cancer, two young mothers – Ruth Picardie and Beth Wagstaff – met and the idea of the Lavender Trust was born. By raising funds specifically for younger women with breast cancer – who often feel unacknowledged by the medical profession due to their age – the Lavender Trust has become a vital new arm to the existing charity, Breast Cancer Care.

'Seven thousand pre-menopausal women are diagnosed every year,' says Ruth's sister, Justine. Beth and Ruth found therapies of the retail and skincare varieties to be the best, and several skincare companies are involved with the Trust. The Lavender Trust has also funded booklets, and due to the Trust's funding, the Breast Cancer Care's helpline is open on Saturdays as well as weekdays. The Trust funds the younger women's breast care nurse, telephone support groups and there are further plans for the future, including a pioneering support group for women with a high hereditary risk of breast cancer, and a web-based chatroom for women to talk to other women in the same situation as them.

Excerpt from an article by Markie Robson Scott
first published in *You* Magazine

A Pioneering Haven for cancer sufferers

A flagship drop-in centre for women suffering breast cancer has just opened in Fulham, following three years of tireless fund-raising. The Haven Centre will cater for women in West London, offering emotional support, a library of information, a range of therapies, alternative therapy services and talks by leading nutritionists.

The services that exist at the moment are scattered and when you have been diagnosed with breast cancer and are going through the treatment, the last thing you need is to have to look for them,' says a spokeswoman for the centre. 'We will be offering alternative therapies such as acupuncture, aromatherapy, massage and hypnotherapy to help sufferers cope with the stress they are experiencing, while boosting their immune system.'

The Centre will also be offering a programme of yoga and gentle exercise classes, as well as organic and macrobiotic cookery classes. Later in the year, the Centre hopes to open a shop selling bras, swimsuits, prostheses and wigs, and will teach women how to use scarves and make-up as an image and spirit booster.

The pioneering centre is the brainchild of former art dealer Sarah Davenport. When her daughter's nanny was struck by the disease three years ago, Sarah noticed that although her hospital treatment was adequate, there was very little support. She raised cash through fund-raising and company donations, and the challenge now is to raise the £500,000 a year needed to keep the centre running, and open more centres up across the country.

Excerpt from an article by Ciara Woodley
Ealing & Acton Guardian

Thursday 2nd March 2000

'The fact is, Rita,' I said one morning, with several newspaper clippings from that morning's post spread out in front of me, 'women get off their backsides and do something about it. Look at all these women who've suffered, and done something because of it. I think it's amazing – we've got Haven Trusts, Lavender Trusts, this cancer centre, that support centre. It's great.'

What also amazed me was that not only were the newspapers and magazines full of articles about cancer and its possible causes, but everyone seemed to know somebody who had recently been through exactly the same illness and treatments. 'This is more prevalent than I ever realised,' I continued. 'Everyone either has an aunt, or cousin, or friend who has had it? A lot of them are women in their forties and fifties, so it's not just the over fifty-five-year-olds who are getting it. This isn't just an older person's disease any more.'

There were even a couple of quite young women. One, who was in her mid-thirties, had been trying for a baby for years. She finally got pregnant, only to discover she had breast cancer. The doctors had taken the lump out and given her radiotherapy, to be followed by chemotherapy after the birth of the baby.

'Did you know that chemotherapy can make you permanently infertile?' I said. 'Thank heavens I've had my children already.'

Rita shook her head in despair. 'I hardly knew anyone who'd had breast cancer when I was your age. Not even many of my friends' mothers had it. There must be something more to it.'

'That's the emerging opinion – they believe many of the cancers developed today are as a result of environmental influences, such as the air we breathe, the cocktail of chemicals on produce to make it look lovely, plump and rosy, to make it last longer, or grow all year round.'

'It can't be good for you,' snorted Rita. 'In my day, fruit and vegetables had a season and we used to look forward to each different season because it brought with it different flavours, and different favourite foods. I mean, not even Christmas has a season any more, with Christmas decorations in the shops in August!'

I laughed. It was true. You could get strawberries at ridiculously early or late times of the year, and raspberries all year round. In fact, I wouldn't even have known what fruit and vegetables were harvested in England in each season. Admittedly, we now import a lot more than we used to, so that also explains why we get a wider variety for longer in each season. But what of all the preservatives they smother them in so they can last the journey without becoming mouldy and rotten? And most of the nutrients are lost the longer they are in storage, transit or in display.

But what was the alternative? Not everyone could have a farm, or even a small holding, in order to grow their own and benefit from eating fresh from the garden. Hell, many of us didn't even have a garden!

'It's criminal!' snorted Rita.

'It's population.' I countered. 'You just have to find your way round the problem. And I'm going to start by making a new plan. I'm going to eat considerably more fruit and vegetables, and I'm going to get round to organising this organic box scheme delivery to my door each week. And in fact, there's also a fascinating article about detoxing, so I'm going to try that, too.'

Friday 3rd March

I rifled through my magazines and found several organic box delivery schemes which I then checked out on the internet. I picked one and placed my order, which was promptly delivered a few days later. I opened the box up, and found an exciting array of fruit and vegetable inside, all seasonal, all fresh and free from herbicides and pesticides.

However, while Rita's praise of seasonality had sounded exciting, I found it difficult not knowing what was about to be delivered in each fruit and vegetable box, and therefore to plan meals ahead as you couldn't guarantee you had all the ingredients. It was also difficult to do the detox diet, as half the fruit and vegetables I needed weren't in the box, so I ended up having to go out shopping, and some of the ingredients weren't even in season. I then faced a dilemma. Should I get the right ingredients to do the detox diet and therefore buy stuff with possible chemical residues, or should I just get what I could from the recommended list of fruit and vegetables and make do with that? Not a woman to do things by halves, I elected to do the latter. If I was going organic, then I was going organic, right?

However, there were several flies in the ointment. The first was Colin's reaction to some of the mustards and sauces I had bought.

'This tastes like shit,' he said, pointing to my new organic mustard one evening at dinner.

I had to agree it did indeed taste a bit bland and earthy. I agreed I would get him some ordinary stuff, but I privately vowed to get used to the taste of it. I was going organic, no ifs or buts.

March

A couple of nights later, Colin took me out for dinner and I realised that I couldn't control what restaurants served.

'No organic restaurants in Kingston,' I said, having trawled through the Yellow Pages.

'Well, eating organic seventy or eighty percent of the time at home will stand you in very good stead.' Colin reassured me.

I also found, to my chagrin, that there were certain vegetables and fruits I didn't even recognise. Sometimes I would hold some produce up and ask Rita what it was, and Rita had to then begin to teach me how to store it, prepare it, cook it, even eat it! I felt like a schoolgirl again, and marvelled at the fact that I had got to the ripe old age of thirty-five without really knowing how to cook.

'But the problem is,' I chatted to my friend Miranda on the phone one evening, 'I don't want just boiled vegetables, particularly as most books recommend you then coat them liberally in butter, which I'm definitely off. Instead, I want to make exciting vegetable dishes, and some evenings to just forget the meat or the potatoes. I want to combine vegetables to make tasty stir fries, or ratatouilles, or whatever. I don't know, because I don't know what the possibilities are.'

'Get a steamer,' advised Miranda.

Another friend suggested I just throw it all together, as all vegetables tasted good mixed. I could add some chickpeas, lentils or nuts for extra flavour. My sister advised me to get some cookbooks.

But when I tried the throwing-it-all-together approach, I conjured up some fairly bland, unappetising meals. No, I decided, there was an art to this – an art I needed to learn.

It was during my recuperation period that I also decided to visit the Haven Trust, the support group in Fulham that I had read about. The environment was cosy and welcoming, with a huge library of books to rifle through. I could see myself spending a lot of time there. They were very friendly and welcoming, and offered me an appointment to chat to their Breast Care Counsellor. I didn't feel I needed any counselling as I had such a supportive family and friends, so I declined.

My quest for knowledge continued. The more people I spoke to, the more I realised I needed to dig deeper. There were certain foods you should eat because of their anti-cancer properties, certain supplements you should take because they eliminate free radicals, whatever they were.

Around this time a girl called Cecilia, the assistant of one of Colin's clients, was diagnosed with breast cancer. She was, like myself, thirty-five when she found out, but they'd identified it in four different places in her body. We chatted on the phone one day about our respective treatments. Hers was far more intensive than mine due to the metastases (secondaries), and she was having both chemotherapy and radiotherapy at the same time as the medical team tried to reduce the size – and presence – of the tumours. She still sounded very shocked, as she had always felt so well.

'I mean,' she said to me, 'it's a bit like caring for your teeth and going to the dentist for thirty-five years, then one day you go and they say all your teeth are rotten and the whole lot have to come out. I've always lived such a *moderate* life – I eat healthily, I exercise regularly but not excessively, I have several glasses of wine a week but I don't overdo the partying or rack up over forty hours a week in the office.'

It didn't sound fair, and I could only sympathise with her confusion and bewilderment. At least I knew I had been burning the candle at both ends for the last eight years, trying to combine a full-time career with full-time motherhood. Cecilia didn't even have children yet, although she'd always imagined that one day she would.

She started telling me all about her forays into self-help – largely, at this point, diet. She had made very radical dietary changes after a week-long stay at the Bristol Cancer Centre, attending their counselling and macrobiotic cookery courses which she thoroughly recommended.

'You need to eliminate free radicals from your system,' she was telling me. 'Free radicals are like toxins in your system.'

'How do you avoid getting them into your system?' I asked, puzzled.

'By eating as many of the right foods as possible.'

Which were? Mostly fruit and vegetables, soya, nuts and beans…

Hmm, I mused. Maybe I should do the Bristol Cancer Centre course, though it would be difficult to leave the children for a week. I was sure they could sense the stress in the house, and it might exacerbate any fears they already had.

Cecilia recommended a nutritionist in London who was very good, though he was really busy so it might take a couple of weeks. In the meantime, I mentioned that I'd read about detoxing and was contemplating it.

'You should,' said Cecilia. 'There are loads around, like the Heart Foundation diet, or the Cabbage Soup diet… they just flush out your system. Any nutritionist or dietician will be able to help advise you.'

But I was unsure. 'I was wondering whether you should do a detox when you're being treated for cancer. Isn't it better not to start meddling?'

'Heavens no. Best time for it.'

'But what if it's the wrong thing?'

'How could it be the wrong thing? They're all healthy diets,' protested Cecilia.

'Well, I read that there are certain foods you shouldn't eat during chemotherapy.'

'Like what?'

'Mushrooms, and citrus fruits… that's all I can remember right now.'

'I never heard that. Some mushrooms you're positively encouraged to eat, like shii-take mushrooms.'

The question was, how did you make sure you ate all the right foods? And how did you know you were eating the right things for you personally – after all, what might be good for one person could be wrong for the next?

Apparently there were tests they could do, such as allergy tests, or metabolic tests. Cecilia gave me the name and phone number of the person she went to see, and I scribbled it down. I suggested we met for a coffee at the Haven Trust, as she frequently went there, and we said goodbye.

We never actually met, and it was quite a shock to me a year later when Colin told me she had died of breast cancer. I cried, partly for her and partly for myself. It really knocked my faith that I would recover from this illness, and I had to talk pretty sternly to myself that everyone's case was individual. Just because Cecilia had died, didn't mean that I would follow the same path.

> *Lesson learned:*
> ### Don't lose faith because of other people's cancer story

I duly rang Cecilia's nutritionist, who indeed was busy for the next couple of weeks. We chatted on the phone, and the woman, Kerry, recommended I see somebody who specialised in terrain analysis, seeing as I wanted to 'personalise' my diet. This turned out to be Alistair Russell, who took various bodily fluid samples from me, then analysed my body's 'terrain'. He spoke passionately about treating illnesses by looking at the whole of the body, not just the part.

'That's the problem with the medical world today. You get head people, heart people, liver or kidney or stomach specialists. But even the Greeks understood two thousand years ago that you need to treat the whole of a person, not just the part.' He pointed to a framed typewritten message on the wall. 'This is my belief,' he continued, beckoning me to read it. It read:

'*(Among the Greeks) eminent physicians say to a patient who comes to them with bad eyes, that they cannot cure his eyes by themselves, but that if his eyes are to be cured, his head must be treated; and then again they say that to think of curing his head alone, and not the rest of the body also, is the height of folly. And arguing in this way they apply these methods to the whole body, and try to treat and heal the whole and the part together... as... the part can never be well unless the whole is well.' (PLATO, CHARMIDES.)*

'And is that what you do?' I asked politely.

'If I'm really honest, the story goes on to say that it's therefore not just about curing the body, but also curing the soul. I personally only seek to cure the body, and I don't get involved in trying to cure the soul,' he answered earnestly.

'How would you begin to cure the soul, anyway?' I asked, so unused to this new world I had entered. My world had always been so full of practicalities, facts and figures.

'See a holistic doctor,' Alistair replied, studying the charts that came up on his computer as he tipped the fluids into a strange mini lab system.

A holistic doctor? My head began to buzz. How on earth had I lived so long, so utterly ignorant that such a different world even existed?

A holistic doctor, he explained, is one who follows what the Greeks called the 'naturopathic' view, rather than the 'allopathic' view that conventional doctors follow. Naturopaths cooperate with the natural healing powers of the body by strengthening and supporting them, and this works particularly well with diseases such as cancer, which is frequently considered an emotional disease as well as being recognised as a dysfunction within the body, where cells mutate and replicate too quickly, thus creating tumours.

Throughout history, differing beliefs have dominated alternately. Hippocratics believed in cooperation with the body's natural healing powers, while others saw this as a mere meditation on death. In medieval times, the naturopathic view revived itself and this was manifested in heating up or cooling down the body to purge it of toxins, then bleeding, giving emetics or applying leeches.

I shuddered as Alistair continued. 'Well, by the eighteenth century, the allopathic view came back to the fore, but knowledge and ability were scant. You might have died in the hands of either school of medicine, but the naturopathic may have been less painful ultimately.' He set his computer to print, and turned round to face me.

'Allopathic medicine took great strides forward with the discovery of antiseptic and pain relief, and painless surgery. It can mend bones, cure so many ills and prolong life, yet it's still recognised that this kind of medicine has limitations with such diseases as cancer. Hence the holistic approach.'

He explained to me that people exist not only on a physical level, but also on psychological and spiritual levels, and all of these must be treated if we are to move forward. Since each person is different, treatment must be personalised to suit an individual's history and family history. So on a physical level, you have nutrition, medicine, surgery and exercise. On a psychological level, the holistic therapist will deal with the patient's feelings, reaction to self and others, and general nature. Spiritual therapy largely deals with meditation, soul-searching and relaxation and, in the case of cancer, visualisation. It can also often take the form of direct action as well. When a person is completely 'spiritually grown', they invariably 'spread the word' by helping others. Spiritual awareness is the common link between philosophical beliefs throughout the ages – the very basis of philosophical debates analysing the relationship between mind and body. Does the body control the mind, or the mind control the body? Certainly the body cannot exist without the mind, but arguably the mind can exist without the body, if the soul is in the mind.

It was all getting very complex and deep. I was relieved when he finally picked the printed pages off the computer which would inform me about the status of my internal organs.

'Firstly, a brief word about Biological Terrain Analysis… this is the study and practice of healing the body by understanding its biochemistry – the amino acids, enzymes, molecules and atoms found within bodily fluids – to find out how it's functioning. We believe we can restore a body to health by monitoring the pH, oxidation-reduction potential and resistivity, and by recommending a diet to introduce a stable environment back into the body.'

'Okay,' I nodded, bemused by his explanation which left me no clearer.

'If you don't supply your body with the vitamins, minerals and nourishment it needs, and instead load it up with processed, chemical-laden food which is typical of western diets today, your immune system cannot function. You become prone to illness and your body can't tackle the illnesses, particularly the serious diseases.'

In my particular case, my digestive system, adrenal gland and kidneys were under serious pressure. Alistair pointed to one chart that showed a picture of the body with red dots indicating parts that were under pressure. 'Your ageing process is good – it shows you as thirty-five, which you are – your circulation and lymphatic systems are good and your liver is okay. But I stress that your kidneys are seriously in need of some tender loving care before the filtering capacity of them is damaged.'

'How do I give them tender loving care?' I asked, imagining myself stroking two small pink slabs of meat.

By detoxing, he told me. I would benefit from mainly eating alkaline-forming foods, and avoiding acid-forming foods, combined with taking supplements such as zinc, magnesium, potassium, trace elements, and vitamins A, D and E.

'Dandelion root is very alkaline forming and great for the kidneys. Probiotics – which are some of the yoghurts that are coming out onto supermarket shelves now – will also really benefit your digestive system.'

'Okay. Will you be giving me this information printed out?'

'Of course. It's all here.' And he pulled forward another stapled sheaf of papers. 'This shows the list of food you should concentrate on, but primarily, as the golden rule, *you must drink more water*. It is vital. Some of this current damage is probably due to you not drinking enough water, and drinking too much caffeine and fizzy drinks. Aim for two litres a day, and consider investing in an alkaline water ionizer. This would really benefit you.'

And what should I avoid? I wondered, trying to take it all in. Maybe it was easier to know what I couldn't eat, rather than what I could.

That sounded easy enough: I should minimise bread and pasta, avoid refined rice, wheat and flour; minimise dairy, all processed and refined foods, all sugary foods, caffeine and salt. Gorging was out – instead, I had to graze on more meals, and not eat later than two and a half hours before bedtime. If I had to eat chocolate, I should go for dark, organic chocolate, and try to make it only every fifth day. Ditto with wine, and it had to be red wine.

'I hope it's all written down,' I said. 'I'll never remember all this.'

'It is.' He handed me several documents. 'Go home and have a really good read through, and if you have any questions, just ask. But understand this. Two thousand years ago, Hippocrates said that "Death sits in the bowel". And modern day scientists have proved that an acid/oxidised cell is primed for degeneration and even cancer, and in your case this is what we need to concentrate on repairing. We must reduce the acid load in your system in order to improve the absorption of critical nutrients from the digestion into the blood and reduce the free radicals in your system.'

'Okay,' I murmured, feeling really quite small by now and somehow as though I'd been naughty, caught eating all the cakes. I said my thank yous, promised to eat alkaline-forming foods and left. I walked out into the street, my notes tucked into my handbag. So much learning to do, complete with a new way of shopping, cooking and eating. This illness had turned my life on its head in many more ways than I could ever have imagined, but I was also feeling buoyant and optimistic as I felt like I was doing something positive about getting better.

I was feeling good, too, about the benefits my newfound knowledge would have for my children. No more processed foods, herbicide and pesticide cocktails. I was educating myself about healthy and nutritional eating in order to protect my children's future.

What I didn't understand, as I said later to my old school friend and next door neighbour, Alice, was why I didn't know this information already. I mean, we had done cookery at school. We should have learnt all about nutrition, but I just couldn't remember doing so.

'No,' laughed Alice. 'We just learnt about mixing cakes. Don't you remember, old Nosey Parker? She used to pick her nose, then come round and test the sponginess of our cakes by sticking her dirty fat finger in?'

'How could I ever forget?' I felt queasy at the memory. 'I rarely ate anything I made at school, for fear of eating something that Nosey Parker had added her special ingredient into the mix.'

'But we only ever made cakes. I don't remember making a single savoury, and certainly not learning about vitamins, minerals, the five-a-day approach to fruit and vegetables,' Alice agreed.

'Neither do I. But I have to say, I do make really good cakes,' I admitted, and Alice acknowledged that she did too.

'Well, we learnt something then,' we laughed.

> *Lesson learned:*
> ***Death sits in the bowel; diet plays a large part in keeping healthy***

I read all the material Alistair Russell had given me before meticulously planning my three-day detox diet. Having this knowledge about the weaknesses within my body strengthened my resolve. I tried to rope Colin and Rita in to detox with me but they both declined, so I steamed ahead with my plan alone.

I went and bought a juicer, as well as the food for the three day process, vowing not to go into a single food shop while I was dieting. I put out a three-line whip on anyone bringing any sweets, cakes, biscuits or crisps into the house, and no alcohol was to be opened. (The latter was easy for everyone else as I was the only drinker in the house).

'I now remember what it feels like to be a baby that's not weaned yet,' I said to Colin that evening, feeling full of liquid.

On day two I didn't even have the morning's kilo of grapes to look forward to. It was just vegetable juice all day, and I was getting sick of cleaning the silly juicer-thing. It was really quite refreshing, particularly the watercress.'

On the afternoon of day two of the detox, I arrived home from shopping with a steamer. Rita raised her eyes to heaven.

'What have you got now?' she asked, examining parts of it as I took it out of the box.

'A steamer. It's important to steam and not boil the vegetables, as boiling often cooks out all of the essential nutrients. You need to eat your veg as raw as possible, hence steaming!' I stood back proudly and looked at my steamer, which to me represented far more than a way of cooking vegetables. This was going to be the gadget that enabled me to improve my digestive system back to full health, thus eliminating the possibility of cancer returning in the future.

'Next it will be all those beans and lentils,' Rita murmured suspiciously.

'No. Those are acid forming,' I said, much to her confusion, and she let it go at that.

Time on a detox diet seems to pass very slowly, all the more so because you try to avoid watching television with all its cookery programmes and advertisements showing succulent lamb chops, or melted butter over a jacket potato. I eagerly awaited meal-times – I'd never known vegetable soup to taste so rich, thick and wholesome. By day three the headachiness had passed and on day four I felt great. So much so that I vowed to do this on a regular basis.

Further reading "Go on… detox yourself"
on the website www.careerkidsandbreastcancer.com

Chapter Eight
Supportive family and friends

March 11th – 12th 2000

I was delighted when my old schoolfriend Miranda suggested she came up to visit with her seven-year-old son. She'd called me to see how I was, and decided to make the journey from Bristol to help me with my struggle on healthy eating. Miranda is big time into alternative health remedies, homeopathy etc. She puts the rest of us 'effluent society' to shame; as my husband puts it, 'Miranda treads lightly on this planet.' She grows a lot of her own vegetables, has chickens, eats lentilly, sprouting things and doesn't burden the NHS as she pays for private homeopathic treatments.

I went out to get some food, fully expecting Miranda & Josh to be late (as usual). But today they arrived when they'd said they would, and we all drove up outside the house at the same moment. 'Excellent timing,' I said, clambering out of the car to meet them. Grace and Eliot hopped around the car door excitedly as Josh unbuckled his seatbelt.

'I brought my Power Rangers,' he said to them, announcing the important news first.

'We've got Power Rangers!' squeaked Grace.

'You've only got little ones,' Eliot admonished her. 'I've got two big ones, Power Ranger Red and Power Ranger Green.'

'Yes, but—'

'Oh, kids! Pack it in, and go inside,' I said, pushing Eliot gently towards the door. I could feel Miranda's eyes boring into me. 'I'm fine. I look pretty normal, don't I?'

She grinned. 'You do actually. I was expecting you to look ghastly.'

We went inside and caught up with each other over a cup of coffee, though we kept getting interrupted by the children. I

suggested a walk around Richmond Park, as it was such a lovely day
– and we might get more peace.

'I find it difficult to say too much in front of the children,' I
explained.

We sauntered across the park. The sky was remarkably clear and
blue, and the weak March sun was just beginning to slant, making
the shadows long. There was no wind, and the cold, sharp air
seemed to have frozen everything into place. Even the grass
seemed frozen, as though each blade had decided that minimum
movement would retain maximum warmth. The sun was certainly
too weak to offer any warmth, only light.

But such beautiful light! The trees, the heather and grass were
bathed in pale yellow, and the children ran happily around, the sun
giving them bright haloes. It was the stuff that picture postcards are
made of, and increased the moment's poignancy. I felt emotion
rising up inside me, and had to physically gulp to push it back down.

'I love days like this.' I murmured, and that's also why I love life.
Oh precious, precious moments.

'They're definitely the best,' agreed Miranda. She saw my eyes
watering. 'Oh, don't fear,' she said, and hugged me, her own eyes
watering.

'But I do.' I surreptitiously wiped my eyes so the kids wouldn't
see. 'Damn! I was feeling so positive this morning. But then you
observe the poignant moments around you, and get all upset again.
My biggest fear is that I won't get to see the children to the age of
eighteen. But then eighteen isn't enough. I want to see them set
their own lives up, travel the world and come back and tell me what
they've seen, fall in and out of love, choose a career, change careers,
get married, have babies… I want to be granny, a great granny…'

'You probably will. You'll probably outlive us all,' said Miranda,
pouring us both a cup of coffee from the thermos. I took it
gratefully, still dabbing away the tears.

'Maybe. Maybe not. But at this point in time, it feels like I have
a death sentence on my head.'

'We all do. We all live every day of our lives with a death
sentence hanging over us.'

'I know. Maybe it's just that I've never thought about death before. I've always just thought about life.'

'But that's great. How positive. I've often thought about death.'

'What do you think about it?'

'That it's pretty final,' laughed Miranda.

'Huh! No, I mean – why have you often thought about death? What is there to think about?'

'Sometimes when I've been ill, I've thought about different ways you can die, whether it's painful or not… whether you really do see lights at the end of a tunnel… if there's life after death, or if you become a fluffy cloud! I've thought about the deaths of other people I've known – my grandparents, the woman in Petersfield who was hit by a train when she got stuck on the level crossing. She was very young, with a couple of children. And it was such a tragic accident, such a waste. What was the point of that?'

'Wow, you *have* had a lot of thoughts about death.'

'That's nothing. I've thought about it so much that I don't really even mind the thought of it now, just for myself, I mean. When I think about death in a wider context, then I'm scared. As you are well aware, when Josh was a baby I was worried about who would look after him if anything happened to me? At that time, we rarely saw his father.'

This made me think. In my case, Colin would obviously look after the children and I was sure he would do a good job, although he needed to be more demonstrative of his love. Men were so undemonstrative, I mused.

'Anyway, if anything happened to you, I'm Josh's legal guardian.'

Miranda nodded, looking down at the ground and saying nothing. *But if anything should happen to me… I thought, understanding her silence.* The ripples of impact of this illness stretched out further.

'Hopefully, Joanna, what will happen is that you'll get your life completely sorted, and have all your contingencies in place, then live to your nineties,' said Miranda, to lift the shroud of doubt that engulfed us both for a moment.

We both laughed. 'But… and this is going to sound really silly, but my mind has analysed lots of silly nooks and crannies in the last few days,' I admitted, blushing slightly. 'I've even started thinking about my pension. Should I invest more into my pension and live on less now… or should I just stop paying into my pension, and spend a bit more now?'

Miranda didn't miss a beat. 'I believe in insurance, so I would pay into my pension,' she said, unsurprised at the workings of my mind.

Suddenly I shivered, and picked up the thermos. 'Let's walk for a minute. I'm freezing. Come on kids! We're going to walk the long way back.'

The children scrambled down from the fallen branch they were playing on. The sun was slanting heavily now, and their shadows made them each look about five foot tall. They skipped and ran, with Miranda and I keeping up a steady pace. When the children had run too far ahead, they paused, drawing pictures in the exposed muddy areas of the path with sticks, and sticking stones into them.

'Look at my picture!' Grace skipped around, as we caught up with them. 'It's a princess, and she has jewels in the crown and dress.'

'Beautiful,' I said.

'And mine's a picture of you, Mummy,' said Eliot. I looked at the wonky circle, with eyes, nose and mouth placed ad hoc in the face.

'Very Van Gogh,' I smiled, wishing I'd brought my camera so I could capture all these precious moments.

In the distance over in the car park, the ice-cream man played his jingle, and the sound carried clearly across the cold air.

'Can we have an ice-cream, please, please, please?' begged Grace. Josh turned to his mother to work on her.

'No!' we both said in unison, caught each other's eyes and laughed.

'It's far too cold, and I've got no money on me,' said Miranda.

'And we're going down to TGI's right now,' I added.

'Hooray!' the children whooped, forgetting about the ice-cream. 'We can have Dirt 'n Worm pie there,' added Grace, and started describing this ice cream & jelly worm feast to Josh. His eyes lit up.

TGI's was dim, warm and extra cosy after our two hours in Richmond Park. It was also fairly crowded in there, so we'd had to split up across two tables next to each other, and in fact everyone much preferred this arrangement. The children were just reaching that age where they relished some freedom from their parents, and parents relished their children's new found desire for independence.

Now the children tucked into their food with relish, having worked up an appetite from running around. Their faces were still pink from the cold. I watched them, a sudden sick feeling in my stomach. Everything suddenly seemed to sharp, so crystal clear, so utterly real. It was as though I had just put on some new glasses which had brought life into sharper focus. Everything took on its own special meaning and importance, things that last week I'd just not seen or not acknowledged.

'D'you know, I go from being positive one minute, to negative the next minute. Death to life, ill to well, sad to happy…' I said, trailing off.

'It takes time to get used to. Not that I know. I've never been given such a bad diagnosis on any of my illnesses, but you must look at the prognosis. They say it's good, don't they?'

'Yes. They do. But are they just saying that?'

Miranda assured me that if the doctors thought I needed to get my paperwork sorted, they would tell me. 'But they're not, are they? What are they saying instead?' she prompted me sternly.

'To wait and see. They have to run loads of tests yet.'

'Just get this first bit out of the way first,' advised Miranda, not having any answers.

Back at home a few hours later, with the children installed in bed, we uncorked some wine. We decided to sit in the conservatory with the doors open, so that Miranda could smoke outside while we still chatted. I turned the heaters on, and we were warm in our sweaters, fleeces and thick socks.

'It's mad, what I'll do for a fag.' Miranda paused, looking at the cigarette. 'I've promised Josh I'll give up.'

I nodded. 'It's one of the hardest things I've ever done.'

I'd had several abortive attempts at it, but in the end it was Colin who'd made me give up when he'd said he loved me too much to stand by and watch me have bits cut off me. I rolled my eyes as I told Miranda this. 'Every conversation I seem to have at the moment comes back to this one subject. Because now I *am* having bits cut off me.'

'*Out*, not *off*,' corrected Miranda.

'Yet, at any rate.'

'You're thinking negatively again.'

'I hated hospital,' I said, a propos of nothing.

'I'm not surprised! Heavens, I gave birth at home just to avoid hospital.' Miranda paused. 'I wish I could say things that make it all better for you, I wish I could say that hospital is fine, that surgeons are great and that anaesthetics are better than any drugs I've ever taken. But I can't.'

This was why Miranda was such a good friend. I'd rather hear her honest opinion than some trite 'doctors are very good nowadays' and 'the hospital you're going to is a very good one' – as if anyone really knew. Mistakes happened, there were bad doctors in great hospitals, and great doctors in bad hospitals. Who was to say whether anyone would happen to get the right combination on the right day?

Naturally the conversation turned to diet – my main pre-occupation at this time, and Miranda is a walking encyclopaedia of food knowledge. She began a litany of information about the additional oestrogens that are pumped into cattle to accelerate growth and milk production… plus the additional oestrogens that are pumped into all the meat, poultry and fish you eat… which in turn as a knock-on effect into all dairy produce – cheese, butter, cream, eggs etc. Then add the oestrogens that are in London drinking water because so many women are on the Pill and are excreting it back into the system. The average glass of water, she informed me, has been processed through the human body seven times over nowadays. Over the course of one week, how much additional oestrogen were we consuming? No wonder, she said, that hormone-linked cancers are on the increase.

Then she launched into her attack on manufactured produce. This is generally high in sugar and salt which damages the liver, as well as possibly having GM ingredients – or the fats being hydrogenated. Hydrogenation, apparently, creates transfatty acids which are very bad for you and have been linked to breast cancer. I showed her the Olivio spread I had been using lately, since I'd heard it was certified GM-free, which Miranda generally approved of as it had no hydrogenated fats and was very low in transfatty acids... mostly vegetable fat. Although five years later I finally came to the conclusion to just use Yeo Valley Organic Butter and forget all the fancy spreads etc. Keep it natural. Keep it real.

Miranda's next onslaught was aimed at all wheat, maize, rice, sugar etc crops as the pesticides, herbicides etc sprayed over crops are a cancer cocktail. The Ecologist has claimed that there are thousands of man-made chemicals being used nowadays, with many of them going untested – and that's with a Government in the UK who supposedly ban any chemicals under the heading 'Known Human Carcinogens'. I argued that they were monitored, and Miranda agreed that they were in this country, but only to a degree. Some of the sprays still used in intensive farming were questionable – which again is proven when in 2005 the carcinogenic Sudan 1 chemical is found in a raft of food brands and has to be withdrawn from our shelves.

Miranda argued that organic farming was not just about the food, but also about the land. Chemicals strip the land of its natural nutrition and natural ecological balance, meaning that give it a few years and we won't be able to grow any crops anyway without chemical intervention, and then where will we be? Consuming more chemicals, poisons and toxins - none of which our bodies can process. We're not even supposed to be meat eaters, let alone chemical eaters. No wonder our bodies get confused, and cells start replicating and mutating when they shouldn't! It is no wonder that *they* believe in fifty years time we'll all get cancer.

"As it is, *they* say that already one in three people will get cancer," Miranda announced finally. "More ridiculous than that is the fact that millions of pounds are spent every year on cancer research – but only on its cure. The real causes of cancer are not addressed."

We chatted on, about diet, lifestyle, and how Colin would think I'd completely lost the plot when he saw the cupboards full of organic mishmash. Suddenly, as we reminisced on the past, a strange thought struck me.

'Miranda, do you remember all those years ago we went to the Psychic Fayre… at Chelsea Town Hall?' I began.

'Dimly, yes. I think I dragged you along, didn't I, because you thought it was all tosh.'

'Can you remember anything I was told that day?'

'Of course not!' she snorted. 'It was at least ten years ago, wasn't it?'

'I know,' I said, 'but I remember. I was told that I had a long lifeline, that it went thin in the middle, which could indicate ill health, and that I had a problem around the left chest area of my body. Don't you think that's a bit weird?'

Miranda nodded. 'Ye-es,' she began slowly, fiddling with the rings on her fingers. 'It certainly sounds, from the snippets you recall, like various things are coming true.'

'I'm wondering whether to see a clairvoyant, or a palmist or something now,' I admitted. Miranda continued looking down at her hands. 'Do I sense hesitation?' I questioned.

She laughed. 'Fact is, Jo, I can't believe I'm hearing such an about-face point of view from you, the ardent non-believer!'

'And?'

'Would you want to know?'

'What?'

'If they foretold death in the next couple of years. Would you want to know?' Miranda said earnestly. 'You're looking at it from the point of view that they say you're ripe for another thirty-five years, but what if…?'

I went silent. Miranda had hit the nail on the head.

'Look,' she said gently, 'I'm the first person who would recommend seeing some fortune-teller if I could see something constructive coming out of it. But I can't see what you would gain.

I think you have far more to gain from looking at the here and now, the today and not tomorrow.'

'But I want something else. Some kind of guarantee… I don't know.' I slumped back in my seat.

'Go and see a nutritionist, explore alternative therapies… there are loads of other options. But do something that's more positive than clairvoyancy. Don't get me wrong, I don't think your time is limited. You're young and strong, you're otherwise incredibly healthy, you have a great mental attitude and you have loads and loads to live for, and you're full of fight. Focus on that, not what some fortune teller might say.'

That night I was restless and barely slept. Information jumbled round my head, swirling madly as I tried to make sense of it all: the facts and figures, the good food and bad food, diets and recipes. I thought I'd learned a lot before Miranda turned up; now I felt like I'd done a degree in Food Nutrition in twelve hours! By morning, I felt in need of a good night's sleep.

> *Lesson learned:*
> **Keep it real.**

Further reading "The GM Debate"
on the website www.careerkidsandbreastcancer.com

Chapter Nine
Planning for the next stage

Thursday 9th 2000 – my 36th birthday

Two weeks after coming out of hospital, I was due to have the stitches removed. It was also my birthday. Normally I let those around me know, organising to go out for lunch at work and making sure Colin didn't forget to book a table in a new, untried restaurant. However, this year I didn't feel like celebrating my birthday or even acknowledging it, and was kind of hoping it would just pass by.

However, Rita had remembered and she'd organised the children into an excited chorus of 'Happy birthday' as I came downstairs. Colin had gone into work early, as he'd be leaving early to meet me at the oncologist later that day. Two happy, excited children sat at the table to greet me; it was already laid out for breakfast, complete with cards and presents. I smiled at them, and realised it had been unfair of me not to have told them. They would have been very upset if they'd missed my birthday, and kids of that age can't even understand dates, let alone remember them.

'Is this all in my honour?' I smiled widely, feigning delight.

'Yes, it's your birthday!' Grace said gleefully. 'You can open my present first.'

'No, mine!' shouted Eliot, pushing his gift into my hands.

'No, mine!' Grace argued, pushing his present out of the way.

'I'll put them behind my back and Rita has to pick a hand,' I said. Both children sat back anxiously as Rita picked the left one. It was Grace's present – some lovely notepaper and envelopes. Just what I needed after all of those phone calls, cards, letters and flowers to wish me well. I needed to write back to a few people.

'I picked it for you,' said Grace, and went on to describe the different selections available and why she had picked this particular one. I sensed Rita's guidance behind the decision and smiled at her.

'And now Eliot's present. I wonder what this could be,' I said, shaking the video-shaped box. 'Shall I try to guess? Maybe it's a pen, to write the letters with? Or maybe it's a new cushion for the sofa?'

'No!' Eliot started laughing. 'It's a…'

'Shh!' said Rita quickly. 'Let mummy open it to find out.'

'Is it a new pair of slippers?' I asked him, and started to unwrap it.

'I'm not telling you!' he said in a sing-song voice.

It was the 'Titanic' video, which I hadn't seen yet. I hugged them both.

'Now you have to open all your cards too.' Grace said, handing her a small pile of coloured envelopes. 'Nanna's been taking them out of the post this week.'

'And after school today we're going to have birthday cake,' said Eliot.

'What a lovely birthday. Aren't I just the luckiest mummy to have two such lovely children?'

> *Lesson learned:*
> **Value life's precious moments.**

I still couldn't drive so my aunt Viv, who lives quite nearby, offered to drive me there and back. Mr Wintry removed the stitches from under my arm, leaving a long red lurid scar that he assured me would fade very quickly. He also removed something resembling cling film that he'd placed over my breast to keep the stitches clean. None of this had actually hurt at all, although I had been pretty nervous about it. And while the back of my arm and armpit were numb, I was not bothered by this. After all, who really needs to have full feeling in their armpit?

After doing all these necessary bits, Mr Wintry inspected his surgery closely then praised my recuperation, saying that I had repaired extremely well both from the anaesthetic and the operation, and he was very impressed with my positive approach, which, he believed, would lead ultimately to my recovery. I felt complimented, but privately wondered whether I merely projected a positive facade. In fact, I frequently felt extremely negative, though I didn't say this to him. Instead, I tried a different tack.

I told him I'd been investigating diet and nutrition, seeking his advice on this subject. He looked instantly sceptical. I added that I'd been advised to go on a detox diet, and all the reasons why.

'How very nice for you,' he said dryly, but expanded no further.

'I just wondered what dietary advice the world of conventional medicine gave to women with breast cancer?' I continued, somewhat officiously, as his obvious cynicism was beginning to irritate me.

'Go home, and live your life like you did before,' he said shortly.

'But that may be what caused the problem in the beginning,' I contested.

'You've done nothing wrong,' he insisted. 'Look, any healthy diet is certainly a good thing, and something that the world of conventional medicine, as you call it, advocates. But don't go mad and eat five pounds of carrots a day. You'll just turn orange.'

Irked, I said that no-one was suggesting five pounds of carrots a day, just a minimum of five fruit or veg.

'That's a Government-issued piece of advice. I hope you didn't pay a nutritionist for that,' he said sarcastically. I decided I'd better end the conversation there before we got into an argument, so I stood up to leave. Mr Wintry observed the abruptness of my movement, and continued: 'Look, I know I'm being cynical, but all the diets in the world are not going to change the outcome for what you have here. By all means, eat healthily, but remember, it's the surgery, chemo and radiotherapy that will cure you in the end.'

'Thank you,' I smiled, not allowing the smile to reach my eyes, but he had already turned his attention back to his notes and didn't notice.

'Now, on a different subject, were you and your husband planning any more children?' he asked.

'No. We were pretty certain that was it. Why?' I replied between gritted teeth.

'Because the treatment can interfere with your cycle, and sometimes even stops it. If that's the case, you may remain permanently infertile.' Mr Wintry said. My jaw sagged.

'Oh,' I said.

'But if you and your husband have finished having your family…' he said, surprised at my reaction.

'Yes, we have,' I said, with less certainty than the first time I'd answered the question. 'A person just likes a choice.'

Mr Wintry continued to make some notes, drawing pictures of my breasts and circling the areas of surgery. I watched him as he carefully drew the two globes, ensuring he'd got the shape right, and I thought how curious the situation was – if a male friend or one of the guys at work sat there drawing my breasts, I'd clobber them!

He must have felt my stare, as he looked up quickly and said he'd like to see me again in four months time. As I left he handed me a book about chemotherapy, which I stuffed into my handbag before making a hasty exit, feeling thoroughly deflated. I was annoyed and upset by Mr Wintry's attitude, but the infertility thing got to me even more.

Lesson learned:
Look for the positive; don't dwell on the negative.

Colin came home that evening to find me looking red-eyed and shifty. 'What's happened?' he asked.

'The treatment may make me permanently infertile,' I said, the tears welling up in my eyes again.

Colin paused. 'Well,' he began uncertainly, 'we've finished having a family…'

'I know that's what we said!' I cried.

Female logic. 'But?' he prodded.

'I want the right to have another baby if I want one.'

'When would you have another one? I mean, if this hadn't happened? We've scraped through the last five years of having babies, coping with the sleepless nights, struggling to afford the childcare. When were you going to have another?' Colin asked, trying to keep the incredulity out of his voice.

'Maybe when I was around forty, before I started hurtling towards the menopause and the decision was permanently taken away from me!' I gulped through my tears. 'Or maybe once your business was up and running, and we could afford for me to stay at home.'

'You'd be bored stupid, and you know it.' Colin admonished. And he was right. I'd always have at least five projects on the go.

'And anyway,' he persisted, 'why? Why would you want to go through all those sleepless nights, the crying, the nappy-changing production line, the endless demands. You were a zombie for three years, Jo.'

I sniffed self-pityingly. 'I know, and I know we discussed what it meant to have another baby around. The fact that we're just beginning to do things we used to do, we can take the kids to Disneyland in the next two or three years. I know all of this. But I didn't want the right to have another baby to be taken away from me.'

'Look, Jo, I could put my arms round you and sympathise, and you could cry and say how unfair it is. Or I could say third baby or breast cancer – which would you prefer?' he asked logically.

We both knew the answer. It was just that the consequences of this stupid illness were so far-reaching.

At that moment the phone rang beside me. I picked it up automatically. 'Oh hi… Oh… oh, that's great news. Yes… oh really?… when was it?… oh, that's great. Mum, I've got to go. I'll call you a bit later when I can talk.' I put the phone down and looked at Colin. 'Kate's just had her baby,' I said, knowing I should feel really happy for her.

He came over and put his arms round me, cursing the timing, but privately thinking how hellish this must be for my mother: one daughter going through hell, facing cancer treatment, the other celebrating the birth of a new baby. She couldn't know whether she was coming or going.

Lesson learned:
Don't upset yourself by focussing on the many small implications of cancer.

Saturday 11ᵗʰ March

The next date on the schedule I had been dreading was my visit to Bill Lucien, the oncologist Mr Wintry had referred me to. I had been dreading this day, as it made the chemotherapy so real and so imminent.

Later that day I reluctantly set off to see the oncologist who turned out to be a friendly-faced older man in his late fifties. Colin met me there, and we walked into the surgery together, both white-faced and wide-eyed. We all chatted for a while about treatment generally, about my surgery, and Bill Lucien enquired about my lifestyle generally before he got onto the specifics.

What he proposed was a course of chemotherapy. In the case of treating primary breast cancer, he told me, they offered adjuvant therapy that is purely to minimise the risk of the cancer returning.

'It's just in case any cells have escaped and gone round the system, but we are not trying to cure the illness, just prevent it.'

'Am I having scans all over, anyway?'

'Yes, we'll do those next week then go straight into chemotherapy.'

To my next enquiry, he told me the chances of finding anything were minimal, and I really shouldn't worry about it. *Easy for you to say*, I thought. After chemotherapy, they would then do a course of radiotherapy – radiation to the local area – again, purely to ensure all the bad cells had been killed off.

I felt that he was talking down to me somewhat. He seemed to be speaking very slowly and gently, although I wasn't really hearing anything I hadn't already heard before.

'What about this Taxol product that's being reported in the newspapers?' I asked.

He shook his head. 'That's not appropriate for you.'

'Why not?'

He looked at me over the top of his glasses. 'It's very technical, but I have chosen a level of chemotherapy that is right for your case. We're not trying to shrink a huge tumour, or eliminate secondaries. This is preventative treatment only, and is treated accordingly.'

'And what can you tell us about HER-2?' asked Colin referring to a new test that analysed the hormone status of the tumour. Bill looked blank.

'I've vaguely heard about it.' he admitted. 'It's very new, and surely you feel more comfortable with the tried and tested.'

'What are the chances of this coming back?' asked Colin finally, having left most of the talking to Bill and me.

'Oh dear, dear, dear. There's no point looking on the bleak side.' Bill turned his bright eyes on Colin. 'Seventy percent of the one in twelve women diagnosed every year survive this disease. Think positively, not in terms of chances of this returning. Your job is to look after this little lady as she has a tough six months ahead of her.' He turned back to me, leaving Colin fuming at his patronising words that contained instructions but no answers. 'You really need to look after yourself, think positively and stop worrying about what could be. After all, if worrying stopped it coming back, I would prescribe it in bucket loads, but it only makes this type of illness worse.'

I felt dissatisfied with this response, but I didn't really know what I had been expecting. We finished up the consultation with Bill giving me his card and telling me to phone him over the next day or two when I was ready to proceed.

But I was having difficulty proceeding with Bill Lucien for several reasons. He was a man, an older man at that, and a general oncologist not a breast cancer specialist. But mostly because he had been my friend Ray's oncologist - and Ray was dead. Whilst the rational part of me understood that Ray's advanced throat cancer was very different from my stage 2 breast cancer, I was still reluctant. It still didn't bode well.

Saturday 11th March, evening

'Conventional medicine's very positive in its promises of cures etc, but it has absolutely no tender loving care side to it,' I moaned to Colin that evening. 'It's just fact, fact, fact and forget the emotions. Complementary medicine seems to be far more caring.'

'It's cure, not care we want,' Colin reminded me.

'It's both actually,' I corrected.

What he found so difficult to cope with was the lack of certainty and information, the constant wait-and-see approach. Despite conventional medicine's more factual approach to cancer, he felt like he was wading through treacle trying to get information. My husband just wanted me to have the best, he wanted answers to questions, but he didn't know how to find either. He felt that the medical world had shut the door in his face by merely telling him to 'look after his little lady'. The best way he could look after his little lady was to be there with her every step of the way, listening to the treatment planning, asking questions to ensure it was the best treatment, making sure his wife wasn't just receiving some post-code lottery standardised treatment. The frustration welled up inside him and made him angry – but anger wasn't going to help.

His mind turned to our friends, Pete and Anna. Pete worked in gene research, and so might be able to shed some light. Colin shut himself in the conservatory and rang Pete's home.

This turned out to be a fortuitous conversation. The outcome of the conversation was a real turning point in my treatment. Pete had worked with many scientists who worked in the field of cancer research, and offered to contact these people to find out who they would recommend for first-class treatment.

'The long-term survival lies in the oncology you receive, not necessarily the surgery,' said Pete, after he had got over the initial shock of Colin's news. 'You need a good surgeon who'll remove as much as he can find, but the future lies in the hands of the follow-up treatment. And it's certainly worth taking the time now to ensure you have information, and that you understand the options ahead of you – delaying the start of chemo by a few weeks to ensure you're proceeding with the person you feel most confident is not going to change Joanna's life in any way.'

'Half the time I don't even know what questions to ask,' Colin said.

Pete's view was that a good oncologist should read the situation. Some patients didn't want to know anything at all; they just wanted to be treated. Others wanted to know everything, and a good oncologist would determine this quickly, and talk to them accordingly. It was also important to make sure you were with an oncologist who was at the forefront of research and development of treatments, someone who had their finger on the pulse. Not all oncologists could offer the latest treatment on trial, and often patients didn't want them to because it comes with a risk. But a good oncologist will always assess the risk factor in comparison to your stage of cancer, and will offer new treatment if and when the time is right.

'For example,' Pete said, 'there's a really new test out now called Her-2… it determines the type of cancer that will dictate the type of hormone treatment Joanna will be recommended. So you want to be with an oncologist who'll test for this.'

'Don't they all?' asked Colin.

'No. It's too recent a development. There are only two places in the country that can run the full test. But leave it with me, and I'll investigate.'

'Have you got time to do this?' Colin asked, not wanting to put upon him.

'Of course, and even if I didn't, I would. I think this is far, far more important,' Pete reassured him.

'I'm sure this guy we've seen today is good, but ultimately he didn't manage to reassure us.'

'Is he a breast cancer specialist?' asked Peter.

'Well, no. And that was one of our concerns, amongst others.'

Pete stressed that I should be with a breast cancer specialist as breast cancer is often hormone linked, unlike many other cancers. Colin thought it might be better to be with a general oncologist, because if they found cancer anywhere else when they did the scans, then surely I would want a general oncologist rather than a breast cancer specialist, wouldn't I?

'No,' said Pete. 'You've misunderstood it. What Jo has is breast cancer, irrespective of what parts of the body it's gone to. If they then find a tumour in her liver, it's not liver cancer, it's breast cancer of the liver because it's known as a metastasis, or a secondary. And you don't have any increased chances of getting any other type of cancer just because you've got breast cancer.'

More of the jigsaw puzzle fell into place.

'I suppose,' Colin asked, 'it makes no difference this oncologist being a bloke? I mean, breast cancer *is* a female issue.'

'It's not, actually. Blokes can get breast cancer although it's very rare. But breast cancers are hormone-linked cancers, and men get testicular cancer, so don't worry about it on that level. However, if Joanna would prefer a female oncologist…'

'Well, not specifically. If the best is a bloke, then we'll have him. We just want the best.'

'What else?' Peter pressed Colin further, sensing there was more.

'Well, I also felt this guy's age was a drawback,' said Colin. He's old, and we don't know where this is going, or how long it will be going on for. Joanna doesn't want to change oncologists because one retires halfway through. Because mistakes happen in hand-over, and one can easily blame the other if something goes horribly wrong.'

'Yes, I see what you're saying, and I would feel likewise although it probably wouldn't be an issue. Leave it with me for a day or two. Don't go ahead with this other guy as yet, and I'll get back to you shortly.'

> *Lesson learned:*
> ***Information, information, information***
> ***Get as much of it as you possibly can.***

Tuesday 14th March

Two days later, true to his word, Pete phoned back and gave me a name. He had spent two days ringing round contacts who passed him onto bigger names in the field of cancer research, and finally he began to hear one name that kept cropping up: Dr Alison Jones at the Royal Free.

'I can't tell you that you should go with her, but I can put it this way: if this was Anna, she'd be going with Dr Alison Jones.' Pete was clearly reluctant to advise me on such a critical issue in case the information was wrong. But his gut instinct, combined with the knowledge he'd gleaned from his various conversations with everyone, told him this information was not wrong. 'I also enquired about your other oncologist,' he added, 'and he also has a good name, so you won't necessarily be making any mistakes by going with him.'

'Yes, but along with the other concerns I have, it sounds like Dr Jones fits the bill best so far – she's a breast cancer specialist and she's a woman.'

So I rang to arrange an appointment, but nothing in life is so straightforward. In order to see Dr Jones, I needed to be referred by my surgeon. So I rang Mr Wintry and spoke to his secretary, explaining that I needed a letter of referral in order to get a second opinion.

'Why do you need a second opinion?' the secretary asked frostily.

I was amazed. 'Because I want one,' I said shortly, not wanting to get into discussion with her about it.

'What's the problem with Mr Wintry?'

'There isn't one. Mr Wintry is a surgeon; I'm getting a second opinion on the follow up treatment, not the surgery,' I said, equally coldly.

'But you've been referred to an oncologist by Mr Wintry. Why do you need to see another one?' the secretary insisted.

'I don't need to justify this, particularly not to you. Can I speak to Mr Wintry?' I said crossly. The line went dead for a while and I wouldn't have been surprised had I just been cut off, but then Mr Wintry came on.

'Hello,' he said cheerily.

I took a deep breath to calm myself back down, before explaining the situation to him. He seemed to take exception to my decision.

'What an awful lot of friends you have, making recommendations on issues they are possibly not qualified for,' he said dryly.

'Yes, I have got a lot of friends, and they're looking out for me. Thank you,' I began, my temper rising. 'I have to say that I'm really puzzled by your own and your secretary's response to this one request. After all, it was you who said in the beginning that I could get a second opinion.'

'That was in the beginning. You have now started your treatment with me, and I work closely with Bill Lucien. It makes it very difficult if you then straddle two different surgery and oncology teams,' Mr Wintry explained. 'What's the problem with Bill?'

'I have no problem with Bill. I understand that he's well respected in his field, but I've been given the name of someone who is a breast cancer specialist, is a female, and I want to see her.'

'Well, it's your right,' he said.

'No. It's my life. I'm not doing this out of rights!' I snapped. 'I'm really surprised… it's not as if I'm getting a second opinion on the surgery.'

'I'll get Susan to fax a letter of referral through to this Dr Jones-whatever's office,' he said in closing the conversation.

> *Lesson learned:*
> **Stick to your guns; this is your life in someone else's hands.**

Thursday 16th March

Two days later Colin and I found ourselves sitting in a waiting room in the Royal Free hospital. It was typical NHS, offering no comfort by way of a smart-looking environment, and the two girls running the desk were clearly overstretched, dealing with several matters at a time as the phone kept ringing. At the same time, staff walked in and out, asking questions and handing them files, and people came in and queued.

I was called through to have my observations done, and was pleased to note that I was right down to nine and a quarter stone. 'I haven't been this weight since before I had children,' I told the nurse delightedly. The phrase clouds and silver linings came to mind.

We were then led through to Dr Alison Jones' office. She was an attractive, energetic-looking woman who was probably in her late thirties, I guessed, feeling relieved. She certainly didn't look ready for retirement in the next ten years. I was pretty sure from the outset that I would be going ahead with this oncologist.

'The surgery you've had looks very good, and I'm glad he got fifteen nodes. I consider that a successful operation,' she began and I felt instantly relieved. Mr Wintry excelled in the operating theatre and that was far more important. 'So you've been to see another oncologist, and now you're coming to me?'

I explained everything to Dr Jones, while Colin sat quietly, letting me get on with it.

'What I really want is to feel informed about what's going to happen. So far I'm getting a rather woolly picture, and just being told to look after myself and not worry. I can't help but worry. I mean, someone's going to fill me with enough poisons to make me sick and make my hair fall out, and I'm being told to sit back and not worry!'

Dr Jones was instantly reassuring. 'Let me tell you what I'm recommending for you. There are six different types of chemotherapy currently available. The weakest one is CMF – although it's still pretty strong – and this is given to much older ladies whose hearts and bodies aren't as strong. One of the strongest is FEC, which I'm recommending for you because you're young and otherwise fit and healthy. You could also have Taxol, but this is generally reserved for very advanced cancers, which you don't have.'

'Okay, I understand,' I said, wondering why this couldn't have been explained so clearly before. There was no great mystery.

'We just have to do an ECG to check the strength of your heart, but I shouldn't imagine we'll find anything untoward.'

'What are the chances of this having spread elsewhere?'

'I'd say very slim. Two nodes positive is still early. After four nodes positive, the risk increases, but we'll scan you all over first. I really don't anticipate finding anything, partly because you're still early stage two, and partly because our machines can't pick up single cells, only clusters. But that's why we do the chemo; it's totally systemic and catches everything.'

'How will I feel?'

'We give you plenty of drugs to counter the effects of the chemo. This includes anti-nausea drugs, steroids to reduce inflammation of the gut, and tablets to prevent mouth ulcers. Chemotherapy basically kills off all rapidly producing – that is, cancerous – cells, amongst others. This includes the lining of the digestive tract, hence the sickness and mouth ulcers; red blood cells hence feelings of anaemia or tiredness; white blood cells, hence a reduction in your immune system's capability and, of course, hair follicles, hence the baldness.'

'Is that all over?' I asked, thinking of my eyebrows and eyelashes. I really didn't want those to vanish.

'Everywhere, except the hair on your legs unfortunately,' said Dr Jones, and we all laughed. 'Sometimes eyebrows and eyelashes get very thin.'

> *Lesson learned:*
> **Chemo-induced hair-loss does not affect the hairs on your leg – this confirms that God is definitely a man.**

'I've heard about ice- caps?' I began.

'Yes. They're very effective at minimising hair loss.' Dr Jones advised. 'They work by freezing the head so the veins and arteries retract away from the hair follicles. This reduces the chances of the chemotherapy killing off the rapidly reproducing cells in the hair follicle.'

'And does it work?'

'On some more than others. And I must tell you that some people find it unbearable - whereas others barely notice it.'

'And what about the radiotherapy?'

'That's local to where the tumour was, and will kill off any cells that may have been missed in the surgery, which is unlikely.'

'Any side-effects?'

'The skin gets a bit red. It's like a very severe sunburn, but nothing more than that. Some people complain of nausea, but that's uncommon, and some people feel tired during it but I'm not sure whether that's just the daily commuting, rather than the radiotherapy itself.'

'Daily commuting?'

'Yes. Radiotherapy will be every day, five days a week for round about six weeks.'

'Well, I commuted for five years to the City. I'm sure I can manage six weeks,' I said dismissively.

'And it's not nearly as much hard work as going to an office,' agreed Dr Jones. We all laughed again before she continued. 'The breast that we treat tends to harden for a while, but will start going back to normal soon after, although it never ages at the same rate as your other breast.'

'So I'll have one droopy breast and one young, pert one by the time I'm in my fifties?' I joked.

'Pretty much,' Dr Jones smiled.

'What interesting times I'm living,' I murmured. 'Sometimes I can't believe all this is happening, but then I get a sick feeling and realise it is.'

'You'll be fine, I promise,' said Dr Jones gently. 'What I propose is that we do the chemo first, as this is systemic, and then the radiotherapy. I also had a fax through this morning from Mr Wintry's office advising that the hormone receptor tests had come back positive.'

'What's that?'

'Whether the tumour is hormone fed, basically. And it is.'

'Is that good or bad?' Colin interrupted.

'Well, it's as good as anything in this situation can be,' she smiled at him. 'At least it means we can treat it with Tamoxifen.'

This, she explained, was a tablet you take every day for five years, which acts like a little hammer in the background, constantly tapping away at any bad cells that might reappear. Tamoxifen was originally a fertility drug, as it sits in the body looking like oestrogen. In the case of hormone-fed cancer cells, the bad cells see the Tamoxifen shape and think it's oestrogen. They attach themselves together, but the Tamoxifen, instead of feeding them, starves them to death.

'I like Tamoxifen,' I agreed. 'I'll have some of that.'

'One thing you may hear is that it can cause other cancers,' warned Dr Jones, 'like cancer of the uterus; but this is extremely rare and we can monitor for that by doing an ultrasound scan when we do the breast scans.'

'Right. I'll have some of that too then.'

'Can you tell us anything about HER-2?' Asked Colin. Dr Jones's eyebrows went up.

'You have been doing your research. HER-2 basically identifies certain types of tumours which can influence the type of treatment - although I qualify by saying that most people have a negative scoring which means that the treatment I've proposed for you is correct. And I'm sure you will have a negative score.'

'Can you run the test?' Colin pressed.

'Of course.' Dr Jones made a note. 'Do you know where you want the test to be done?'

'Yes, at Dundee University.' and Colin handed over the name that Pete had given him. Dr Jones nodded in approval

'Any other questions?' asked Dr Jones.

'What could have triggered this?' I asked hopefully, but Dr Jones shook her head.

'We've made some great strides in cancer research, but there's still a lot we don't know. There are certain people who we can pinpoint as being in a high-risk category, but you're not one of them. Give it another twenty-five years and we will have gone beyond looking at the genes, and start understanding what triggers different gene action.'

'Whereabouts are you up to in the study of genes?' asked Colin, genuinely interested.

'Well, we've now gone beyond the genes themselves, and we're looking at the proteins to understand the catalyst actions – what prompts a cell to do what.' Dr Jones explained.

'It wouldn't necessarily have been a hard bang to the breast then?' I asked.

'No. A hard bang can trigger certain cancers, but not breast cancer.'

I had to ask. 'Is it the food I eat?'

'That's a big theory going round, and we cannot say definitively no. You may have eaten something that had carcinogenic sprays on it, or unknowingly lived near a nuclear station that leaked or something. But nothing, in terms of diet, has been clinically proven. However I always encourage my patients to investigate their own cures in conjunction with mine, as long as they tell me what they're doing.'

'Could it be stress?'

'Stress weakens your immune system, and certainly would have made it difficult for your body to deal with. That's one of the reasons we recommend people don't work during their treatment, as we need to build the immune system right up again. That, and the fact that not many people feel capable of working.'

'Okay. And what are the chances of this coming back?' Colin asked finally, wondering if Dr Jones too would just fob him off. But she answered.

'Without treatment, there's a 30% chance; with treatment, about 15%. But these figures are misleading, and you can't really apply them to an individual, so having told you those figures, I now urge you to not dwell on them, because there are other factors to take into consideration. Time is one of them. The chance of it returning is higher in the first five years, and this decreases over the next five years. After ten years, we can effectively sign you off our books as you then have the same risk factor as anybody else of developing any type of cancer.'

'And if it does come back?' I asked anxiously.

'Then we start on the next cupboard of treatment. We do a mastectomy, followed up by a course of treatment that may differ from this first course of treatment. Added to which, we scan you regularly over the next ten years in order to catch it very early.' Dr Jones was very forthright in her answers.

'What are the statistics?' Colin pressed her.

'Well, Tamoxifen has saved 30,000 women's lives over the last five years, and like I said before: you've found this early, and breast cancer is the most treatable. I promise you, I will look after you.'

'Thank you. I need looking after,' I said gratefully.

'You'll be fine, I promise. If you have any feelings of sickness, then I'm not doing my job properly.'

I looked at Colin, wordlessly seeing if he agreed that I should proceed with Dr Jones as my oncologist. He nodded. 'If you're happy,' he agreed.

I nodded back and agreed to go ahead with the treatments, then signed on the dotted line.

> *Lesson learned:*
> **Just keep asking questions;**
> **a good oncologist will have the answers.**

Further reading "Patient's guide to Chemotherapy"
on the website www.careerkidsandbreastcancer.com

Chapter Ten
The next leg of the journey

Friday 17th March

Dr Jones' secretary, Teresa, rang me the next day, making appointments to have me scanned from top to toe at an imaging centre in Wigmore Street and have a heart scan at The Royal Free. More incremental processes in the long journey towards cancer cure.

'Dr Jones said they're not expecting to see anything on the scans,' Colin had tried to reassure me that morning.

'Only because the cells might be too small,' I said negatively.

Monday 20th March

I sat on the train as it sped its way towards Waterloo. Ordinarily, I mused, I would be at my desk having my second, maybe even third cup of coffee. Phones would be ringing; at the desk opposite me, Kerry would be talking loudly down the phone, and Jenny across the room would be clicking busily away on her keyboard, not to mention the occasional slamming down of a phone from Jane's desk. But instead I'm here, on a train hurtling towards Waterloo to be x-rayed. These x-rays may provide information about my body that I'm currently blissfully unaware of, but information that could tear my world to pieces even further. Do I want to know? Would I rather just carry on not knowing? Just live in ignorance until this illness, or maybe even another illness, comes and takes me? Obviously not. I asked Dr Jones to throw the book at me, and that's what she was doing.

> *Lesson learned:*
> ***In your bid for complete cure***
> ***take what is on offer, then ask for more.***

I'd been told countless times that it was learning they had cancer that often caused deep, introspective evaluation and huge lifetime changes in sufferers, and invariably it was for the better. One girl even went as far as to say that her friend who'd had breast cancer had said it was the *best* thing that ever happened to her! Hello? I could not get behind that one at all. Whichever way I looked at it, I couldn't see any redeeming features of breast cancer, and could think of many better events in my life – and few worse. Perhaps with many, many years' hindsight, *after* you had survived the cancer ten years or so, then maybe you would be able to see some positive changes you'd made to your life following diagnosis. However, nobody had made a guarantee at this stage that I would make it to another ten years, despite my oncologist being pretty certain that I would, and giving me every indication that what I was suffering from now was eminently treatable in this day and age. But what if the cancer cells just decide, *boom*, I'm going to carry on doing my worst. They might be particularly aggressive, or whatever triggered it in the beginning might just carry on triggering. How could I actively prevent it coming back without knowing what had triggered it in the beginning? That was doing my brain in. If only… if only somebody somewhere could just say: this is why you got it. Because whatever it was, I would give it up. Even if it was something difficult to avoid or give up, I would anyway. I shook my head in frustration.

And what would I be re-evaluating anyway? I'd always known that I loved my children, my husband, my family, my house, my lifestyle and my job – I had learned nothing new in the last three weeks about any of those key aspects of my life. So what? Maybe I had started opening my eyes a bit wider about my lifestyle, but nothing that was hugely impacting on my day-to-day life.

I was still deep in these thoughts when I finally looked up and realised I was already in Wigmore Street. I found the address and was sent straight to Reception. After some form-filling, I was given a chalky, milkshake substance to drink – in huge quantities – before being called through.

I spent the next few hours being shunted through various huge circular machines, or being draped around x-ray machines as they tested my body, my bones, my back, my head, my womb etc for further evidence of cancer. I found I was becoming increasingly numb to the potential possibilities, partly because I'd experienced the worst of the shock with the original diagnosis, and partly because I had come to finally accept that what would be would be, and worrying would not solve the problem. If it had already spread, then it had already spread. I was having the chemo and radio therapy now anyway, and if the cancer had spread, they would just give me more, and in more places. They said put your arms up, I put my arms up; turn this way, and I turned this way; that way, and I turned that way. I was on auto-pilot, just obeying instructions as they were given.

After several hours and many x-rays, I left with the advice that I was mildly radioactive and should avoid cuddling my children tonight. I wondered what reason I could give the children, because certainly they would not understand the truth. More importantly, I also left with the information that they hadn't seen anything yet to give cause for alarm, but the plates would show more detail and I could contact my oncologist on Friday to get the definitive diagnoses. Well, at least they couldn't see anything major, I told myself as I made my way back home.

I got back on the train the next morning and met Pete at the client's office. We told the client that I would be off work for a while and that I was handing the project over to Pete and a project manager, Jason, and I explained briefly why. The client was very sorry to hear the news and wished me all the best. Afterwards, Pete and I went for lunch where we ended up demolishing a bottle of wine, and I felt really quite tipsy when I left to go to the hospital.

'We need to take a blood test first,' said the nurse, showing me into a room.

'Oh. Does it matter that I'm a bit drunk?' I asked guiltily.

'Did you drive here?' asked the nurse.

'No,' I said, puzzled.

'Then it doesn't matter,' she said, and I laughed.

The heart scan involved lots of little pads being stuck onto my body, which stuck to my skin via a conducting gel. It was time-consuming and I had to sit in some uncomfortable positions, but the guy doing the test said that I had a really healthy heart.

'So they found nothing,' I said to Colin that night.

'Not even your heart?' he asked lightly.

'Ha, ha! They found no cancer tumours anywhere. And they said my heart was 100% normal.'

'Excellent,' said Colin, getting out a bottle of champagne that he'd had chilling. It was, he believed, important to mark the high points of this whole process.

> *Lesson learned:*
> **Celebrate all the little bits of good news along the way.**

Tuesday 21ˢᵗ March

The next couple of days passed quietly. Colin and I had both explained to the children that Mummy was about to start a course of medicine that would make me very tired, possibly sick and probably bald. Grace and Eliot had both laughed nervously at that thought, then Eliot protested, saying that he preferred mummy with her long hair. I assured him it would grow back.

On Dr Jones's recommendation, I had a hair appointment on Tuesday to have it cut short, really short, shorter than I'd ever had it before in my life. I pulled a face at myself in the mirror as I scraped my hair back, trying to visualise what I would look like bald, but the image just did not appear. The darkness of my hair made it impossible to see. I stood brushing my hair and styling it for a long time the evening before. I liked my hair, it had always been long and thick, and I didn't want it short – and I certainly didn't want to be bald! But now it was all about to go.

As it turned out, my friend Terri-Anne did a really lovely haircut. It was short, but not so short that I felt naked. I still had a thick mop of hair on my head, and the shortest it got at the back was to the nape of my neck, and everyone said how much it suited me. Eliot still wasn't convinced as 'Mummy has always had long hair'. Grace was more tactful, saying that she thought it looked very pretty but she preferred mummy with longer hair.

I had spent the early part of the week meeting friends for lunch, and generally trying to achieve a relaxed and calm sense within. However Thursday was looming, and I was feeling increasingly nervous and anxious.

'Just the thought of it makes me sick, I don't need the actual chemotherapy to do that,' I joked to one friend at lunch on Monday. It was the thought of a nurse injecting me with toxins, watching them flow into my body and knowing that it would have such severe after-effects.

Wednesday 22nd March

On the Wednesday, I went up to the Haven Trust again and saw some small posters advertising a talk that was happening in two weeks time. It was about the link between diet and cancer, by a nutritionist called Suzannah Olivier. They were expecting it to be very popular, so recommended getting your name down early. I put my name down, and made a note in my filofax.

I went over to the library where I found a promising book about protecting your body from cancer, which I borrowed and went home with. It was fascinating, and I spent the afternoon curled up on my bed reading the book eagerly. By the time Colin had come home, I'd read it and was bursting with new information.

I told him all about it, and was surprised when he poo-poohed it. 'Nobody controls what happens at cellular level in your body. You can't do anything to make sure your cells breathe aerobically or anaerobically,' he scoffed.

'Well, clearly you can, according to this book.' I pushed it into his hands. Colin took it and read the back cover.

'The guy who wrote this isn't even a doctor or a research scientist,' he said, looking at me in bewilderment. I was lost for words. 'He's just a bloke who's spent years researching and collating other people's findings and thinks that a fruit diet will save you! I would trust Dr Jones's judgement rather than this guy's. If Dr Jones says they haven't found a cause yet, then I would go by that. After all, she's a research scientist and a qualified oncologist who, according to the medical profession, is one of the best.'

I started pointing out some of the facts that the author had listed, and argued that this guy couldn't just be making it up.

'I'm sure he's not. I mean, this point about lactic acid – that's what muscles produce when you go on a marathon. You've heard the term "hitting the wall"? Well that's when your muscles can't cope, lactic acid fills the muscle area and you start screaming in agony – it's a warning signal to stop. If you don't, you then get beyond the pain and can carry on running and running. I don't see where the link is to getting cancer.'

'All he's saying at the end of the day is what everyone else is saying,' I said, trying to defend that which half an hour ago had seemed to be an 'answer'. 'It's about having a healthy diet.'

'Great. Well, you're doing that. And you've done the detox thing, that's great. But don't go reading this stuff and tell me this guy knows the answer to how you can avoid getting cancer. If he really did, he'd be worth a fortune and nobody would be suffering from cancer!'

'I don't see why you're so negative about him,' I pouted.

'Because the whole premise of the book seems to be inferring that it's *your* fault you got it in the beginning… your fault because you ate the wrong foods, and your cells started breathing incorrectly, and your blood sludged up because you ate too many fattening pies,' Colin said crossly, then turned to me, putting his hands round my face and saying earnestly, 'For pity's sake, this isn't your fault, and there's nothing you could have done to stop it. I wish you'd stop beating yourself up over it.'

I paused before realising he was right, then hugged him tightly.

Lesson learned:
It's not your fault… cancer is an extremely complex illness and rarely has just one cause.

My mother rang to offer to collect the children on Friday night. I was about to say that I was fine, when I remembered thinking that I'd been 'fine' before I went into hospital and look what happened then. I was feeling really stressed and nervous at the thought of chemotherapy, and really not in the frame of mind to consider anybody, not even my children.

'Maybe it would be a good idea,' I agreed and Mum was relieved. She'd been convinced that I would struggle manfully on, refusing to acknowledge how fundamentally my world had just changed; that nothing was wrong, or that it wasn't that serious, and that I could manage just fine. But one look at my face would tell anyone I wasn't fine. I'd lost a stone in one month, I was sheet-white and had dark shadows under my eyes which I'd never had before, despite my usually heavy workload. Many people marvelled at how I seemed to have the strength to keep on living my life normally, as though none of this had happened. But my mother didn't marvel out of admiration. She marvelled out of fear, as she feared the day that this illness, treatment and their impact suddenly hit me.

> *Lesson learned:*
> **Despite what modern-day women are led to believe…**
> **you don't have to be super-woman.**
> **Take the help where and when it is offered.**

After putting the children to bed, I ambled through to the sitting room and the kitchen, looking around me and seeing the cosy untidiness of children's toys, my papers and various bags, shoes, jackets etc that collect in rooms when a family really *lives* in its house. But I could not be bothered to tidy up. Colin was working late tonight, as he was accompanying me to the hospital the next day, so I had only my thoughts for company. I walked through to the conservatory, stepping over more toys and things on my way, and stood aimlessly at the French windows, looking at the garden that was looking rather wintry and bleak. The trees were bare as everything had been cut right back in November in order to encourage spring growth.

I cast my mind back to November. God, I'd been so utterly unaware of the bomb that was coming my way. I felt the tears start running down my face again. 'I don't want this medicine! I don't want this treatment!' I hissed at the garden, my breath steaming up the glass in front of me, knowing that whatever I thought of it, I would be going through it anyway.

Further reading "Analysing cancer closer"
on the website www.careerkidsandbreastcancer.com

PART TWO

Chapter Eleven
First step on the road to recovery

Thursday 23rd March

On the morning of my first chemotherapy, Colin had to go into work early to finish off something critical. I said I would take the train to the hospital if he could meet me there with the car, so he could drive me home afterwards.

Now I was sitting on the train as it hurtled its way between stations. It was odd to think that this was a journey I'd undertaken many, many times before as I commuted between work and home – the daily grind and irritation of being jostled by the crowd as everyone fought for space on the train and battled their way down the steps to the tube. Today, I also struggled with my nerves.

'I'll be fine,' I muttered to myself, as I trudged down the tube steps with five hundred other commuters. 'And this, truly, is an unpleasant start to any day, wherever you're going,' I thought, looking at the people milling around me and remembering why I had left my previous job. A large part was to get out of the commuter traffic. It was an insult to expect people to herd around like sheep.

'The hardest thing about coming to work,' I used to say as I arrived at work, 'is the actual *coming* to work. *Being* here is the easy bit.'

By the time I arrived at Belsize Park, I felt crabby, tired and grubby. I walked up the hill and round the corner to the Royal Free Hospital. Inside, millions of people buzzed around, doctors with stethoscopes and implements, nurses with notes and plastic bags of specimens, trainee doctors and nurses with clipboards or folders, people on their own, people in large crowds. It was mayhem.

I was told to go straight to the 11th Floor where I was to have my 'obs' done. They weighed me – nine stone! Wow! I had lost weight again. They measured me – five foot seven. Phew! I hadn't shrunk. They then went to take some blood from me.

'What's that for?' I asked.

'We have to do it before giving you chemotherapy,' the nurse said, surprised.

I held out my arm reluctantly and turned my head away.

'You'll get used to it,' the nurse said, rubbing the vein with antiseptic.

'Why's that?' I asked, trying to keep my mind off the moment the needle went in.

'Sharp prick,' said the nurse unnecessarily. 'Because you have to have a blood test every week now.'

'Every week? Until when?' I squeaked, trying to not move suddenly with a needle sticking in my arm.

'Well, the end of the chemotherapy. How many… Are you alright?' the nurse asked quickly, seeing the colour drain from my face.

'No, I'm not. I hate blood tests,' I said faintly, bending forward to put my head between my knees and breathe deeply.

'Are you going to faint? Get some water,' she instructed another nurse.

I sat up and took the water as it was offered, seconds later. 'No I won't faint. I just feel faint. I have very low blood pressure, and blood tests often make me feel faint. I didn't know I had to have so many, either,' I added.

'We need to keep an eye on how your body's responding to the treatment, but the girls in the chemotherapy suite will explain everything to you,' the nurse said quickly, fearing she'd said too much already. She put a little round Elastoplast over the needle prick, and sent me downstairs to the tenth Floor Chemotherapy Day Room.

There was no one around, and I had to guess where to go. On the tenth floor I followed the wide corridor to the left and saw a sign saying Oncology, so figured I must be heading in the right direction. I passed three rooms in a row, each one with recliner seats in them occupied by people who were hooked up to drips.

Doctors flitted around, and a lady with a trolley was going round offering tea, coffee, biscuits or sandwiches.

Everyone flitted past me, so finally I collared a man in a white coat, introduced myself and said why I was there.

'Can you take a seat there for a moment,' the doctor said, looking vaguely harassed. I sat down, thinking 'Come on guys, make this easy on me otherwise I'm running.'

'Hi, I'm Elaine,' said a Scottish girl coming over, with a clipboard. She checked my name and date of birth. 'I'm going to be looking after you, and Dr Jones will be up shortly once we've you settled in,' she smiled, and I felt relieved that someone was taking control. Colin arrived at that point, and we were both taken into the Chemo Suite, Colin looking as grey as I felt.

Elaine took me to a recliner chair and made me comfortable, making small talk as she did so. I was offered tea or coffee, but elected for water. They also gave me a tuna sandwich which I never ate. Dr Jones came in to see me, and they ran through some fine details about the treatment. They were going to set up the drip with saline solution in it, and leave that running for a while to flush out my veins. In that time they would also put the ice-cap on, which was changed every half an hour. After the first half hour, they'd start administering the FEC, which would take around forty-five minutes.

'We have to do it slowly,' explained Dr Jones, 'so that the chemicals don't burn the inside of your veins. If you feel any soreness or burning, tell us immediately and we'll stop. Sometimes the canula can pop out of the vein. Also, before the treatment we'll give you these anti-nausea drugs, and these are also some introduced intravenously.'

'Which are the steroids?' I asked suspiciously, looking at the little pot of pills.

'The white rectangular ones,' said Elaine.

'I don't like the idea of taking steroids,' I admitted.

'They reduce the inflammation in the lining of your gut, and will help prevent nausea,' said Dr Jones.

'I read that they make you put on weight, and I don't want to end up like a body-builder.'

'They can do,' admitted Dr Jones. My heart sank.

'But then again, I also read that they can shrink tumours,' I said, more hopefully.

'Indeed, but as far as we know you don't have any now.' Dr Jones patted my arm, not patronisingly but warmly. 'You may put on a bit of weight with them, but you'll lose it again straight afterwards. Don't worry,' she added, understanding my reticence.

'I'm so nervous,' I whispered, feeling the tears stabbing my eyes.

'You'll be fine,' Dr Jones rubbed my arm. 'Honestly. I'm not just saying it.' She turned to Elaine and requested that I was given a couple of sedatives, which were duly added to the pot of tablets.

I took the tablets, and the drip was wheeled in. Dr Jones left, and Elaine returned with a trolley. I stared at it suspiciously, but everything was covered up. I watched dumbly as Elaine put on some surgical gloves and began opening up sterile bags with needles and cotton wool balls, pots of antiseptic liquid and the like. She put the needle into my forearm, stabbing around a tiny bit before pushing it in fairly deeply. I didn't want to watch, but morbid fascination kept my eyes glued. Elaine took the needle out and affixed the line in with tape, before fiddling with a little wheel on the drip and blood went back up the line an inch, then back into my body. I felt sick with nerves and from watching the proceedings, but my head was beginning to feel heavy and muzzy from the sedatives.

'I'm just going to go through this little book of information on chemotherapy,' said Elaine, as another nurse came in with the ice-cap. I was told to sit forward, which I did with some effort now that the sedatives were taking effect. The new nurse put a plastic shower cap thing on my head, then a neoprene swimming hat that was freezing cold, following by another neoprene swimming hat that was much tighter – more like a neoprene riding hat. My eyes and forehead froze instantly, so the nurse pushed some paper towels up underneath the hat to cover my ears and forehead. I felt like my face was pushed into a frown, but I was floating now so I didn't particularly care. Colin said something about how charming I looked. I grinned and tried to focus on him, but my eyeballs were going everywhere. Lovely, lovely sedatives.

Elaine was running through a list of instructions of what to do, expect etc that evening, but her voice came to me in waves. I heard Colin laugh, and by agreement Elaine then issued the instructions to him instead. I struggled to keep my eyes open, but knew I wasn't hearing a thing.

'Will you give me the book?' I slurred finally. Elaine and Colin laughed.

'I don't think this is making much sense to you at the moment is it?' she said smiling.

'I'm very cold,' I muttered.

'I'll get some blankets for you,' said Elaine getting up. I felt the blankets being draped over me which gave instant and welcome warmth.

Time became meaningless. I snoozed, feeling waves of abandon washing over me, every now and again opening my eyes. Colin was sitting on one side of me, desperately trying to keep light-hearted conversation going with Elaine, who was sitting on the other side of me, looking down at my arm in concentration. When I followed her gaze, I saw Elaine had a huge syringe in her hand which she was slowly injecting into the tube. A thin red ribbon of chemicals fluttered along the tube and into my arm. I closed my eyes and turned my head. Someone came along and put a new ice cap on my head, just as the first one was warming up and becoming bearable. I felt them struggle with my drugged, wobbly head, but I was beyond helping them.

'Let me sleep,' I mumbled, as the caps were pulled and tugged onto my head. I looked down at my arm and saw Elaine was injecting yet another huge syringe full of chemicals into my arm – a clear liquid this time. I shut my eyes and let myself get dragged off into the other world. It would be over soon, I thought, as I drifted off again.

Colin watched all of the proceedings, feeling sick and overwhelmed. He had moved his chair from beside to opposite me, as he found it difficult to stop his eyes from wandering round the room to the other patients, sitting patiently in their chairs with their drips drip-dripping into their arms. Most of them looked so skinny and pale, so bald and so ill. It ripped at his guts that his wife was going through all of this… that she would become one of the grey-faced, bald people he saw in this room. Unfortunately, when he moved his chair, he was then directly facing his wife and then he couldn't stop himself watching Elaine injecting the chemicals into her arm. He wanted to leap up and shout '*Stop*! Don't put that stuff in her!' But he couldn't. He knew it was for the best, but every muscle in his body was screaming to get them to stop.

'How's it going?' he said, as I opened my eyes and looked vaguely at him.

'I'm very cold.' I muttered. He draped another blanket over me. I snuggled down into the blankets and shut my eyes again as Elaine carried on slowly injecting the chemotherapy drugs into me.

Next time I woke up, Elaine had gone and the drip had been moved away from me. I looked down at my arm and saw that the canula had also been removed, but the heaviness of my head told me I still had the ice cap on. It was weird to think that all those drugs were now inside me, poisoning my system, killing off cells as they raced through my body. I mentally probed my body to see if I had any side-effects yet.

'Ah, you're awake.' said Elaine appearing in front of me. 'I think two lerazapan are maybe a bit much for you. You're quite sensitive to them.' She smiled, and I shook my head to clear the muzziness.

'I'm desperate for the loo,' I said, throwing off the blankets and trying to stand up.

'I'm not surprised. You had nearly two pints of saline solution through the drip,' she smiled, catching me as I got unsteadily to my feet. 'Here, I'll take you.'

I weaved my way out of the room, frequently banging into Elaine, and saying sorry every few seconds. She took me into the loo, and I grabbed the handrails.

'Any problems, pull the red cord,' said Elaine clearly, showing me the red cord as though I were an idiot.

I nodded as she shut the door. I looked at myself in the mirror, and laughed at my scrunched up face under the tight hat. 'Truly lovely,' I said to my reflection, before swaying out of sight of the mirror.

I managed to go to the loo, and make my way back into the day room. 'We'll take that off shortly,' said Elaine. Colin smiled at me, thinking how funny I looked in that get-up.

'Before you go, I'll give you a bag of medicines and blood test forms. Have your blood tested at your local GP's each Friday, then get them to phone the results through to us. Take your medicines diligently – they'll keep you from feeling awful.' Elaine carried on listing instructions, but try as I might, I couldn't make sense of it. Elaine looked at Colin, and he nodded to show that he had acknowledged what she was saying.

When it was time to leave, I thanked Elaine and weaved my way downstairs, propped up on one side by Colin. I was better able to stand now, but just felt rather tired, light-headed and light-limbed, as though I couldn't control my arms and legs properly.

'How was it?' asked Colin once we were in the car.

'An injection, a drip, an ice-cap and some sleep – and very cold,' I murmured, my head lolling back on the headrest. Colin put some quiet music on and drove home in silence, with me snoozing away beside him.

I couldn't really remember getting home, but suddenly I was home. Colin opened the front door and I stumbled in, picked up a bottle of water from the kitchen and went straight up to bed, where I promptly went out like a light.

Daylight streamed in through the open curtains, and I woke up unable to tell if it was late afternoon or early morning. I sat up, shook my head to clear it and had a glug of water. I looked at the clock – it was five o clock. It must be 5pm, I decided, on the same day. I had no idea how long I'd been sleeping or what time I'd got back home.

Downstairs, Colin was sitting in front of the computer in the conservatory. 'How are you feeling?' he asked.

'Like a space cadet,' I said and went into the kitchen, looking around aimlessly. I hadn't eaten all day and was feeling starving hungry, but as I raked through the fridge and the cupboards, nothing tempted me. Knowing I must eat healthily now, I opened the fridge and got out some lettuce and tomatoes, deciding to have a salad.

I was sitting in the conservatory, gazing mindlessly out into the garden and eating my salad, when the phone rang. Probably Mum wondering how I was, I thought. It was, and I explained what had happened to me that day, trying to make light of it. Why does one do that? I wondered afterwards. 'I'm now just sitting here waiting for the reaction… for a whirr or a click, or a bang to go off somewhere in my body,' I joked.   Mum laughed, more politely than humorously.

'Is Colin with you?'

'Yes.'

'That's good. Well, if you want to give me a call later, you know where to find me.' She said before saying goodbye.

Colin ran through the list of tablets, and together we wrote out the timetable of what I was supposed to be taking and when. It was quite a comprehensive list – some every four hours, some three times a day, some before each etc etc etc.

I sat mutely in front of the television for a couple of hours before deciding to go back to bed at about ten o'clock. Colin said he'd be up shortly. But exhausted as I felt, I barely slept all night and by the early hours of the morning I had a pounding headache which wrapped around my head in a tight band. I rang the hospital, who recommended Migrileve if I had it, which I did – I'd had so many migraines in the last year that I had packets of Migrileve stashed away in cupboards, bags, desk drawers etc. They also pointed out that I should not have taken the steroids that night, as I'd been so dosed up with them during the day.

'It says on the pack not to take them after 5pm as they can cause sleeplessness. And you didn't need to start the course until tomorrow,' the on-duty doctor told me. I felt silly, and spent the night pacing around restlessly before finally crawling back into bed at 5.20 am to go to sleep.

Friday 24th March

I slept in late the next morning, having vaguely been aware of Colin leaving much earlier, and him saying to call him if I felt ill at all. Rita had already got the children up, dressed and off to school, so the house was silent when I woke up. After taking my tablets, all in all I felt okay and spent most of the day reading. Apart from my stomach and guts feeling very painful, I didn't actually feel sick, just a bit light-headed and disconnected – I couldn't really be bothered to make the effort to talk to anyone. Apart from taking calls from my brothers and sister, who all rang to see how I was, I left the answer phone on and kept a list of the kindly enquiries from friends and work colleagues so I could call them back when I felt up to it.

Rita brought the children home from school at about 3.30 and made them their tea. Mum appeared late afternoon with quite a few shopping bags. 'Just a few supplies,' she said, stocking up the cupboards and fridge. 'Now. Would you prefer I took the children home and left you here on your own to sleep over the weekend? Or would you just prefer that I stayed here?' Mum asked, leaving no room for any other alternative.

I knew that if the children stayed, they would be demanding attention the whole time, asking for food and drinks and 'can-you-help-me-with…', and that I would feel obliged to get up and do, or feel guilty watching my mother running around.

'Do you mind taking them back to yours?'

'Not at all.'

'Yes. I think I'll rest up better if the house is silent.'

'Right. Well, I bought a whole load of bits of food – pre-prepared snacks and meals to make sure you eat up. You've lost far too much weight.'

'You shouldn't have,' I said gratefully. 'Thanks a lot.'

Mum shrugged it off, wishing she could do more, and more, and more. This felt like the least she could do. She took Grace upstairs with her, and Grace helped to pack their clothes for the weekend, which Grace felt very important doing. They all stayed for tea, after which Mum bundled the children into the car and I waved them off.

The weekend passed by quickly and very quietly. Colin and I generally pootled around, Colin watching over me to make sure I rested. Generally I hate resting. I get all twitchy and fidgety, and need to get up and *do* something, but something in Colin's manner told me I'd better get my head around resting and learn how to do it. I didn't set foot outside the front door once, but just sat around reading and watching television and videos, in between snacking on all the food Mum had loaded into the fridge. Being an expert and experienced mother, she had bought loads of crackers and things great for nausea like Grisini sticks, so that I could just munch on them to take the metallicky taste out of my mouth. I found myself falling into a nervous, dreamless sleep during the afternoons for around three hours, and would wake up feeling anxious, unrested and heavy-limbed, and therefore still able to climb into bed at around 9 pm and fall virtually straight to sleep in front of the TV in my bedroom.

Mum brought the children back on Sunday evening, and we spent a quiet evening together. Colin told the children that mummy was *very, very* tired as she'd had a *lot* of medicine. He didn't want to frighten them, but wanted to impress upon them how good they must be, and how helpful they must be to Mummy right now. It had subdued them, and I feared he'd stressed it a bit much, but Colin dismissed this fear, saying that my health and state of mind mattered far more at the moment, and the children had to learn that they had to look after their mother as well as vice verse. It was a family issue, after all, and not to be hidden from the children.

'How's it all going?' Mum asked me.

'Fine. I haven't felt too sick actually, although the lining of my mouth is crumbling. It feels horrid – really rough and as though it's going to break out in a million abscesses.'

'Have you got tablets for it?'

'Yes, and I'm taking them. I phoned the doctor who suggested I also try an antiseptic mouthwash, which I'll buy tomorrow.'

'You should have told me and I could have got it,' said Mum reproachfully.

'I'll need to get out tomorrow. And I really don't feel that bad.' I said.

Famous last words. I walked into Kingston the next day to go to Boots, and found I had not got the energy to walk back home again. I had to sit down on a bench for half an hour until I'd summoned up the strength.

'Okay. I don't feel that bad as long as I don't do anything,' I admitted to my sister on the phone that evening.

'I told Anne about your illness,' Kate said, referring to an old schoolfriend of hers. 'I hope you don't mind.'

'Not at all,'

'Well, she's got a friend who has an apartment out in Argentiere near to where Anne lives, and she's just gone through chemotherapy and radiotherapy for breast cancer – although I think she had a mastectomy. She said she would happily talk to you if you want someone to talk to…'

'Yes, it helps to talk to other people, to compare notes,' I agreed. 'Although I'll probably meet people in England…'

'No, this girl Sarah lives in England – she just goes out to Argentiere on occasion.'

'Oh I see, then yes, I'd definitely call her.'

Kate gave me the number. 'What are you going to do all week?' she asked.

'Potter. I'm going into the office tomorrow, just to say hello.'

'Do you want to come down here?' Kate asked hopefully.

'That's an idea. I could do, couldn't I? I could see my new niece.'

'Yes,' said Kate, pleased. 'How's Thursday, for you?'

We set the date and hung up. My calendar was filling up quickly with seeing friends in-between various medical appointments, which was good. I seemed to think only about cancer, and every conversation was punctuated with thoughts or comments about the illness, the treatment, the impact of it or whatever. It was in my head 24/7 whether alone or with friends, but at least friends & family always added new perspectives which made me feel like I was getting closer to understanding what was happening in my life.

Tuesday 28th March

I don't know what it is about my health but I'm appalling at judging how I feel. The trip to the office exhausted me more than I anticipated. I had arrived there just before lunch. Everyone inquired after my health, whereupon I said I was fine – what really can a person say? – and answered questions about projects I'd left weeks earlier that other people had helpfully stepped into the breach to complete. I noticed that everyone was stretched to the limit now that they'd absorbed all my workload as well, but I couldn't exactly feel guilty!

Then a thought occurred to me. Though I felt faint and giddy after just half an hour in the office, I was bored at home so I offered to take some work home with me.

'The chemicals only affect my body, not my brain,' I joked as I extracted a presentation from Pete that needed writing. 'I'm bored stupid and need something to do.' He relinquished it gladly. I got home, put the papers on the table and went straight to bed to sleep that awful dreamless, twitchy sleep for a few hours.

The next morning, I walked into Kingston for a nice relaxing facial. I told the beauty therapist about my cancer and the treatment, and the girl said she would make sure she would use very gentle, relaxing aromatherapy oils. I lay back, closed my eyes and relaxed. This was just what I needed, and not only for the relaxation: my skin was beginning to look an awful shade of grey and I had big purple shadows under my eyes, so I needed something to put some colour back in my face. I also hovered outside the gym, wondering when I would feel up to doing some exercise, but even the thought of it wore me out. Another time, I decided. There was no rush.

Thursday 30th March

In between sleeping and relaxing with the children, I worked on the presentation. My brain relished the challenge, but physically it wore me out. I was relieved when I managed to get the first draft through to the office for Gina to start laying out. That had broken the back of the thinking and planning, which I had no doubt my boss and colleagues would be thankful for.

On Thursday, I set off for Kate's after the children had gone to school. It was a lovely day, unusually sunny for that time of year, and it bolstered my spirits even further. I was already feeling high on the fact that the chemotherapy had not made me sick, or excessively tired. I'd had no severe reaction to it at all, and I wondered what all the fuss was about.

We went for a walk in the winter sunshine, down to the park with Kate's new baby, Cosima, and her other daughter, Sophia. As we strolled we chatted about life, work, kids, and the conversation naturally came round to the subject of chemotherapy and infertility.

Kate told me that a friend of hers had found out she had breast cancer during her first pregnancy.

'How awful!' I said. 'What a blight on what should be such a happy time.' I looked down at the contentedly sleeping baby, and thanked God I'd already had my two children before the illness struck. 'What happened?'

'They did a lumpectomy during the pregnancy, and then did the chemotherapy after the baby was born.'

'Can you have a general anaesthetic during pregnancy?'

'Apparently yes. There's an anaesthetic that has molecules that are too big to cross over into the placenta.'

'And what about future babies?'

'I think she had one of her ovaries removed and frozen to protect future eggs, so she could have a new form of IVF.'

'Heavens! What a procedure.'

'She's been remarkable throughout, actually. She's just finished the chemotherapy recently, and is really very positive about the future.'

'You have to be.' I agreed. 'But I wouldn't want another pregnancy now, even if I was fertile. All those hormones rushing around your body could be enough to kick it all off again.'

'Could it?' asked Kate.

I didn't actually know, I admitted; I was just guessing, because mine was a hormone-receptive cancer.

We sat silently for a while, watching Sophia cycling around the park on her bike, playing with some new found friends. I cradled my new niece in my arms. It was another of those poignant, precious moments.

'What's the chemotherapy like?' asked Kate.

'Not as bad as I thought, actually. But they say it has a cumulative effect, and that I'll probably find it harder and harder as it progresses.' I described what had happened when I'd had the chemotherapy. Suddenly, I became very aware of little Cosima's weight and began to feel very tired. 'Shall we go back now?'

Kate looked at me, remarking on how drawn I looked.

'It seems to be the way it goes. When I run out of energy, I run right out. It's like running out of petrol, with no reserve tanks.'

> *Lesson learned:*
> **Chemo drains you of energy – a bit like a car running out of petrol. It happens quickly and unexpectedly.**

We ambled back up to the house, where I lay down on the sofa for an hour while Kate prepared lunch for us, and fed the baby. After some bread and soup, which also helped to recharge my battery, I took my tablets and made sure I drank plenty of water. I was still consciously trying to get my intake up to two litres a day, which seemed a huge quantity in comparison to how little I usually drank.

Around three, Kate set off with Cosima to collect Isabel, her oldest daughter, from the school up the road, leaving me with Sophia. I suggested she left the sleeping Cosima behind as well, after all, it would only be for twenty minutes.

'She's too young. I'm still at that stage where I can't have her outside my view for even a few minutes,' Kate confessed. 'It would be like leaving my arms behind, or something. I hate it when people cart her off. I know they usually mean well, to give you some peace and quiet, but I go chasing after them to get my baby back.'

'I remember that. Particularly at a social gathering. One moment your baby is at your feet, sleeping in the car seat, and suddenly the car seat's empty!'

We both laughed at ourselves, at our paranoia and foibles. 'But what the hell. It's my baby. I'll get as protective as I want,' Kate said defensively.

I left soon after Kate got back, wanting to avoid any rush hour traffic. She promised to come to Kingston to visit another day, later on in my treatment, as it had been a rare treat being able to just sit and chat, without the constant interruption of four children that accompanied our usual time together.

It had been a lovely and rare day together. Whilst we had talked about the practicalities of my illness and its treatment, neither of us needed to verbalise how each other felt about it. A knowledge borne out of a lifetime of being close.

Friday 31ˢᵗ March 2000

On the Friday morning, I dutifully took myself off for my blood test following the first chemotherapy session. The oncology team had organised for these blood tests to be taken at my local surgery, rather than me trekking all the way to the Royal Free each Friday which was rather a relief. Blood test done, I left and forgot all about it, and instead spent an enjoyable weekend with my kids, marvelling at how well I felt in comparison to how unwell I had expected to feel.

Tuesday 4ᵗʰ April 2000

The second week following chemotherapy passed calmly. My older brother, James, was over from Hong Kong on one of his fairly regular business trips, so he, Colin and I went out for dinner to our usual haunt – the Chinese restaurant down the road from his flat in Putney. It never fails to surprise me that James voluntarily goes to Chinese restaurants in England, as I would have thought he would crave anything but! We had a lovely evening together, and I was pleased that James was due to be in England on a monthly basis for the next 6-8 months. So I had plenty of opportunities of spending more time with him.

Wednesday 5th April 2000

On the Wednesday, I went to the Suzannah Olivier talk at the Haven Trust that I'd put my name down for. It was really interesting, and I found myself gaining deeper levels of understanding about health and nutrition. It wasn't just about eating organic food, but also reviewing the whole balance of what food groups were on your plate. I bought Suzannah Olivier's book and spending a couple of days reading that, I spent a fair amount of time fiddling around in the kitchen learning how to cook new, healthier recipes.

This also meant having to buy even more specialist cookery books – how to cook the different vegetables, how to make a wide variety of juices, how to steam your food, recipes with nuts, beans and pulses. Some of my offerings were initially quite dire, but Colin was patient and allowed me to use him as a guinea-pig. Some evenings he would devour the lot, whereas other evenings he picked at the food before admitting defeat.

'Don't do that one again,' he'd suggest with a half-smile, half-grimace, and I would get up and mark a cross in the corner of the recipes that were a dismal failure.

Tuesday 11th April 2000

Towards the end of the second week I was feeling less tired and ended up going into the office a couple of times because I really didn't know what else to do with myself. Knowing how frantic everyone was in the office, I volunteered to do a couple more new business proposals as well as specifying and overseeing the creation of a job tracking system for the business. Also the Directors were pitching for a new part of the business with one of my existing clients, so I went to a meeting with the senior global management team who were surprised to see me there, knowing my condition, and told me to make sure I didn't overdo it. I protested, saying I felt fine and promptly spent the next two weeks working on the proposal, presenting working drafts then developing it further.

Everything was going swimmingly, and I felt confident that the chemotherapy was not going to affect me too badly despite all the public scare-mongering about how vile it was. I dutifully went off for my blood test on the Friday, and spent the third week after chemotherapy dividing my time equally between office and home, and sleeping and working. I was beginning to feel a bit tired, but my brain was racing and I had loads of excess energy to burn off.

It came as a surprise when Dr Jones called me on the Tuesday, two days before my second chemotherapy was planned, to tell me that my blood test results indicated that I was reacting quite badly to the chemotherapy – my red and white cell count were very low, and I had to go on to antibiotics immediately to prevent the risk of an infection. They were putting my chemotherapy back by a week, and would require a further blood test on Friday to check I was okay to press ahead. I was devastated, and started crying on the phone.

'I thought I was doing so well,' I said to Dr Jones.

'You are. This is a really strong mix we're giving you. I'm only giving you the antibiotics as a preventative measure, and I'm sure you'll be up and ready to have session number two next week. But you must promise me to take it really easy. This is critically important, as cancer cells grow when the immune system is low.'

I thought guiltily about how I had spent the last ten days, and realised that I had to let go of work for the time being; in fact, by doing any work now and tiring myself out, I might do irreparable and possibly fatal damage to myself.

'What I'll do,' continued Dr Jones, 'is after the next chemotherapy, I'll give you a course of injections which help to rebuild the red and white blood cells. You just have to take these for five days, starting on the fifth day following chemotherapy. You can either go to your doctor's surgery for them to give the injection, or you could do it yourself if you're feeling very brave.'

'No way,' I said, trying to imagine me sticking a needle into myself. My heart was sinking enough at the thought of more needles being stuck into me – it was bad enough having a blood test each week.

> *Lesson learned:*
> **Don't work. Focus on learning how to relax.**

I completed the proposal I was working on, then took it into the office to Pete. I explained that I wasn't doing as well as I'd thought, and that it was probably best if I did not take up any further work for the time being. He was, of course, completely understanding, and suggested I just go home and try to find myself something relaxing and creative to fill my mind with, instead of trying to jam facts and figures into my brain.

One of the girls from work, Jenny, came over for a drink one evening to see how I was and have a chat.

'I just don't know what to do. I'm sitting around with my brain racing but my body is incapable,' I moaned to her.

'You're supposed to be recuperating,' said Jenny.

'Yes, but how do you recuperate?'

'Get a hobby, like painting – pictures not walls – or sewing, or something. Something gentle and creative, and something that's an end in itself, not a means to an end. I'd hate to come back and visit you next month to find ten gainfully employed machinists set up in your back room, churning out cushion covers or something, and you poring over profit and loss sheets,' teased Jenny, and I laughed at myself.

11ᵗʰ – 19ᵗʰ April 2000

So in the third week following chemotherapy, I worked very hard at trying to relax, to do nothing. I read books, practised my culinary skills, watched television, and played quiet games with the children, including teaching Grace to sew which she actually quite enjoyed she ended up sewing a little purse for Eliot as well. The enforced inactivity generally drove me up the wall with boredom, leaving me with unburnt nervous energy, but it must have done me some good because Dr Jones signed off my next blood test, and I was deemed fit enough to have the second round of Chemo. *Good and bad, good and bad,* I told myself.

Further reading "Achieving a healthy lifestyle"
on the website www.careerkidsandbreastcancer.com

Chapter Twelve
Homeopathic support

Thursday 20ᵗʰ April 2000

I woke up early, dreading today. My second chemotherapy. Urgh! Although it's not so bad, I kept telling myself. I was shown straight into the chemotherapy suite as Dr Jones wasn't coming to the Royal Free today.

Whereas last time they had put the needle in halfway between wrist and elbow, this time they went into a vein further down by my wrist as they cannot inject into the same place twice. I had a fleeting thought about how difficult it must become if you have to have many, many sessions of chemotherapy. I should consider myself lucky that they only had to find six places! Fortunately the nurse got the needle into the vein first time, so they didn't have to make a second attempt.

The sedative started working, and I let my head rest back on the bed. The procedure was pretty much the same as before, with a second nurse appearing every half an hour to put on a freezing cold ice-cap, and me occasionally opening my eyes to see huge syringes being emptied into the drip that led into my arm. I was relieved when I felt the nurse removing the canula, and heard her mutter something about getting my tablets and injections while I wore the ice cap for a further forty-five minutes. I snoozed again before being woken by Carolyn removing the ice-cap.

'Thank heaven for that. I hate that thing,' I said, huddled under several blankets.

'You'll warm up quickly enough,' she smiled. 'Now, I've brought all your tablets and injections up as well. Dr Jones has recommended a course of injections called G-CSF which should help to rebuild your system. I've brought them with me today as I want to ensure you know what you're doing, but normally you need to pick them up from the Pharmacy downstairs.'

I nodded, my brain only half working. Carolyn saw my eyes roll in my head, and figured she was wasting her breath. 'On Day Five… counting today as Day One… you start this course of injections. It's one injection a day, injected subcutaneously… that's into a fatty area of your body… for five days. Either you can do it yourself, or your local doctor's surgery will send a district nurse to do it. Okay?'

I nodded sleepily again, trying desperately hard to listen and concentrate. Fortunately, Colin walked in at that moment, and introduced himself to Carolyn. 'Thank heavens,' she said lightly. 'I'll tell you what she's supposed to do with these injections.'

From my drugged perspective the session was finished as soon as it was started – and I was free to go.

Having woken once at 1.35am, rather disorientated, I fell asleep again and slept straight through the night, probably because I hadn't had the extra steroids this time. The traffic and activity on the road outside finally roused me at eight the next morning.

I felt woolly and fuzzy, but not sick which surprised me. I'd always heard that sickness went absolutely hand in hand with chemotherapy. The chemotherapy drugs kill of all rapidly reproducing cells, which is basically the cells from your mouth to the digestive exit point – aka your arse – hence the feeling of sickness. Removing the top layer of the digestive tract leaves the system pretty sensitive! The lining of my mouth felt like it was ragged and pitted with holes. It was horrible but the tablets Dr Jones provided me with were designed to minimise this damage, so I became religious about taking the tablets.

> *Lesson learned:*
> **Take the tablets offered to the timetable specified.
> They really do work.**

There was some post on the mat, and I collected it en route to the kitchen, where I had a leisurely breakfast and spent the morning reading the papers and generally lazing around. My mother rang to find out how I was, and we arranged that I would drive down to hers on the Saturday, stay Saturday and Sunday night, then drive back up on Easter Monday. That jolted me into remembering Easter eggs, which I had not bought yet, so I took a gentle walk into Kingston that afternoon.

Stepping outside suddenly emphasised my feeling of disorientation, a bit like when you've just had a bad flu and have gone outside for the first time for four days. My head felt miles above my shoulders.

Colin called me on his way home from work at around five o'clock.

'Wow! You're early,' I said, surprised. Normally he was at work until eight or nine.

'It's Easter, we've been working bloody hard, and we've decided to all leave early and enjoy the four-day holiday,' he said.

'I'm glad you've remembered it's Easter.'

'Why?'

'Because of the chocolate, silly. It means you've actually remembered to get me an Easter Egg this year.'

'Oh right,' said Colin, guiltily. He never equated chocolate with Easter, unlike his wife and children. To him Easter meant a four-day weekend. 'But you don't want chocolate. You're on a health kick.'

'It's not a health "kick" – that, sonny, is a whole way of life, not some four-month fad. Do you think I would invest so much time trying to change my whole approach to food and cooking for a fad? Nope. You'd better get used to it, because this is for ever.' I warned him teasingly.

'Good. Then you never want chocolate again.'

'You're allowed treats, particularly on birthdays, Christmases, Easter, Valentine's Day and Mother's Day. And I'm having such a bad time at the moment that I don't just want one measly little egg. It's gotta be huge.'

'You'll get fat,' he warned. Half an hour later he walked in the door carrying several plastic bags.

'Here's one… two… three… four. Four Easter eggs, you fat cow,' he said, setting them out on the table in front of me.

'Oh, Happy Easter to you too,' I said, looking happily at the mountain of chocolate in front of me, before giving him a little chocolate heart.

23rd April 2000 – Easter Sunday

The children woke up in an excited state as I always abandon my usual rule of No Chocolate Before Lunchtime, and all eggs and chocolate treats are just put out on the table. Between Mum, Kate and me all buying chocolates, the children had loads to keep them quiet, and Mum planned for a late lunch, knowing that everyone would be full up.

Monday 24th April 2000

On Easter Monday we had to leave early as I had to meet the district nurse back at our house by 10.30am to have my first injection. I told the children to stay in the sitting room while the nurse and I went into the conservatory. After much form-filling, Marion administered the injection into my upper arm. After so many blood tests and intravenous needles, this injection seemed tame in comparison. It was only an hour later, when I felt completely drained and my eyesight went blotchy, that I decided this injection wasn't as tame as it initially appeared.

Colin took the children out to MacDonalds for lunch so I didn't have to cook anything, and we let them watch videos all afternoon. I just lay on the sofa feeling completely exhausted, and half-heartedly managed to get the kids into bed by eight-thirty.

Tuesday 25th April 2000 - am

Tuesday was not much better, particularly as Colin was back at work. I dragged the children round to the doctor's surgery, where Grace promptly hid her eyes against my arms so she couldn't see the injection. Eliot, on the other hand, gawped in morbid fascination. On the way back they pestered me to stop at the playground and I, guilty at the memory of their afternoon in front of the television the day before, complied. I sat down on a bench, huddled up feeling cold and blotchy again, and watched the children run around. *Just keep on running*, I willed them, hoping they would tire themselves out so they could play quietly at home all afternoon.

It was grey and overcast, not a hint of Spring in the air despite the lateness of Easter this year. Nearly May, the end of Spring, and the season seemed barely in its infancy. There were no daffodils around yet, and we'd only had a couple of sunny, Spring-like days. The church clock struck ten, and the day stretched before me ominously. I wasn't going to last another five days looking after my two energetic children, and I had vowed that I didn't want them to suffer as a result of my illness or treatment. I decided I'd phone Rita and see if I could take her up on her offer of having the children.

Eliot called me, wanting to be pushed on the baby swing, and I reluctantly stood up and walked slowly over to him. I lifted his solid little body but had to put him down again, not having the energy. I breathed deeply, flexed my muscles and tried again. After a bit of struggle, and draining every bit of energy out of myself, I managed to get him into the baby swing, then stood there pushing him, feeling quite faint.

'Hello!' said a cheery voice on the other side of the fence. It was Jean, the mother of one of Grace's schoolfriends.

'Hi,' I waved feebly. Jean came in with her two children, and Grace squealed delightedly at seeing her friend Megan.

'How are you?' asked Jean, herself the picture of health and energy.

Feeling faint, I clung onto the frame of the swing. 'Feeling ghastly,' I admitted as Eliot asked to get out of the swing. I struggled to lift him.

'Here, let me do that,' Jean said, taking over quickly, and Eliot ran off to join the two girls on the roundabout. 'Can I do anything to help at all?'

'That's kind of you. I'm actually going to call Rita and see if she wants two little visitors for a couple of days up in Waltham Abbey, as I have to say, I'm feeling exhausted and don't think it's fair on the children if I just keep loading yet another video in.'

'Well, let me know if she can't. In fact, why doesn't Grace come over to ours today, and that just leaves you with one child to manage? I would offer—'

'That would be lovely, if that's okay with you,' I interrupted. 'It makes an enormous difference having just one child rather than both. Are you sure?'

'Yes, if she wants to come over.'

'I'm sure she would. Grace!' I called, and Grace looked up. 'Do you want to go to Megan's today?'

'Oh yes!' squealed both the girls. Eliot stopped in his tracks. He didn't want to be left out, so I bribed him with ice-cream and a video that we would watch together. I was feeling so tired – but still not sick – and during the afternoon I rang my mother-in-law and asked if I could bring the children up to her for a few days. She willingly agreed.

Tuesday 25th April 2000 - pm

Both children were delighted to go to Nanna's house, and apart from a slight reluctance on Eliot's part to let go of my arm, I left quite quickly without any fuss. I drove home slowly, doing fifty in the slow lane on the M25 but I still managed to have an accident. I think this was the beginning of my brain beginning to suffer. The accident happened in a traffic jam with people inching forward. I moved forward far enough and hard enough to smack into the car in front and damage his boot to the point it would not close again. I don't really understand how it happened. How could I drive into him in a traffic jam? I wasn't looking away – I just totally misjudged the small distance. To this day I'm still puzzled. It's as though I lost a critical three seconds of my life; my eyes and brain just didn't connect.

The other driver and I exchanged details, and I set back off again, trying to concentrate really hard. I was relieved when I finally arrived home. When Colin came back I told him what happened. He wasn't bothered about the car (being a rather big and solid Freelander, it showed no signs of having been involved in an accident anyway), but he was worried about me driving around if the drugs were affecting my judgement.

Tuesday 25th April 2000 - night

I had an awful nightmare that night. I was at work, and had to leave to pick the children up from school but it was difficult to get out of the door. By the time I arrived at the school, the last few children were trickling out and their classrooms were empty. There were no teachers around, and nobody I could ask. I ran home, hoping to see my children outside the front door, hoping that maybe Grace had had the presence of mind just to go straight there – but no. There was nobody there. Where were they?! I looked round in a panic. My dream clipped, like a film does, to Grace and Eliot. They were walking through Kingston town centre, Eliot crying because he wanted his mummy, and Grace saying that Mummy was at work, and they would walk to my office and find me, and she was sure it was this way… or was it?

In my dream, Grace and Eliot looked so lost, so small and so vulnerable walking through the town centre on their own. Somehow, I understood that they were in Kingston and started running into the town centre. I ran the whole way, my body screaming for oxygen, my voice screaming their names.

I woke up, breathing heavily and fast, as though I *had* just run into Kingston, and my heart was banging in my ribcage. My hands trembled as I reached across for my bottle of water and drank deeply. When I lay down again, I stared into the darkness, trying to banish the dream, but by the time I got to sleep again, the sun was rising and the dawn chorus was twittering outside.

Wednesday 26th April 2000

I felt awful the next day, and rang Dr Jones to talk to her about how badly I was sleeping. She asked if I was having nightmares which surprised me, but she said it was common when the steroid dose was too high so she reduced it.

'Are you actually being sick?' she then asked.

'No. I just feel drained of energy."

'Well, we're doing everything we can insofar as the injections are concerned. The only other thing I can suggest is getting some homeopathic advice. A lot of my women do that, and some of them really swear by it.'

I was sceptical about homeopathy. I had been in touch with a homeopath, who had said she couldn't really do anything to help as chemotherapy drugs were so powerful. But Dr Jones was recommending it, and as far as I was concerned, she was God and her word was law.

I called the number Dr Jones had given me of a homeopath called Alison Hamilton-Bailey who was based in Barnes.

'Hi, I don't know whether you can help me,' I began. 'I'm going through chemotherapy at the moment, and wondered what homeopathy could do to help me.'

'Well, certainly I can help. With cancer generally, and certainly with chemotherapy, the liver and kidneys tend to get very stressed, so we would look at detoxing them to ease their burden,' Alison advised.

'Oh I see. Can you measure what my liver and kidneys are doing at the moment then?' I asked.

'Yes. We'll put you on the machine, and the good thing about that is, you can be regularly checked and it helps to show you what good you are doing to your body by regular detoxing and healthy eating.'

'Do you help cancer patients often?'

'Oh yes. Some practitioners fight shy of treating the side-effects of cancer or its associated treatments, but I've got many clients who have come to me because of their cancer. What type of cancer have you got?'

'Breast cancer.'

'And was there anything in particular in your treatment that you're having a problem with?'

'Only the tiredness, a feeling of air-headedness, restless sleep and bad dreams.' I listed.

'Come and see me on tomorrow. We'll have a good chat then, and look at how your body's coping with the treatment,' Alison said. We agreed on a time, and I wrote it in my calendar, knowing that if I didn't do it immediately, it would pop right out of my mind. I was really becoming quite vague and forgetful.

Thursday 27th April 2000

Having always been cynical about homeopathy / alternative / complementary medicines, I was in two minds about the visit to Alison Hamilton-Bailey, the homeopath. What could it possibly do for me? I asked myself. Plenty, I answered many months later.

Alison asked me loads of questions, and I told her what I was going through. We discussed it all in great detail, then she put a band around my head which measured all the electrical impulses that went from various parts of my body to my brain. It was connected to her laptop via several wires, and I had to sit with this contraption on for about twenty minutes, while she studied the computer screen.

'Mmm. The ear labyrinth is coming up?' she said questioningly.

'I had a bit of a cold last week,' I admitted, 'and my ears always block up very quickly.'

'Oh right. That explains that then. Jolly good. What else? Your kidneys are quite good…'

'Oh really? That's good, because I was told a month or two ago that they weren't in very good condition, but I've been drinking loads of water and green tea since then. And really cut down on alcohol.'

'It's paid off then, because they look fine. Your liver is fairly weak, your thyroid is good but your metabolism's a bit jumbled – chromosome six is coming up, which is a breast cancer chromosome.'

'Oh! Does that mean I've still got some breast cancer cells in me?' I panicked.

'No, it means that we can treat it with a remedy which sorts out the metabolism jumble,' Alison said quickly. I was still puzzled, and her explanations did not clarify my confusion, but my brain was definitely struggling with concepts that ordinarily I would grasp quite quickly. She continued: 'Your adrenal gland is under a lot of pressure, that needs sorting out. But all in all, I would say it's pretty good for somebody going through chemotherapy.'

Alison took the band off my head and I stood up to look at the pictures and data on the screen. They didn't make much sense to my seized-up brain.

'So what happens now?' I asked.

'I'll give you some remedies, and a list of other remedies that you'll need to phone a company in Ireland for, but they'll send them to you fairly quickly. Take those and I'll see you in a month.'

She disappeared for five minutes, then returned with some little packets.

'This, SOL, is for breast pain, it just helps mend the scar tissue. Take it once a day. The NATMUR is a constitution remedy to be taken once a day, and the CARCINON helps the immune system – take these for the first few days, then one once a day for a month. And take the BERB, which is a kidney flush, once a day – just a drop in brandy each evening.'

'In brandy? Oh what a shame,' I said dryly.

Alison smiled. 'Most people accept that quite readily. And this is the list for liver and adrenal liquescence and METAB for your metabolism. That should rebalance everything. Come back in a month and we'll put you on the machine again.'

'Great,' I said, taking the packets and the letter, and making a mental note that I might well bring Grace to see Alison about a couple of things.

Colin, of course, was amazed at the packets and potions he found in the kitchen that evening. 'Have you checked all this with Dr Jones?' he asked, and I explained that Alison Hamilton-Bailey came on Dr Jones's recommendation.

> ### Lesson learned:
> ### Homeopathy can help counter the effects of treatment for cancer, but cannot treat cancer in itself.

During the course of the week, I made sure I rang the children morning and night at Rita's, hoping they weren't beginning to feel 'passed around', but equally knowing they were having a much better Easter holiday at their grandmother's than they would have had if they'd stayed at home. And with that thought I had to content myself. I went off for my jabs each morning – and the blood test on Friday morning – and divided the rest of my time between reading, eating and sleeping. My sleep was restless and anxiety-filled, and I would wake up feeling upset and twitchy.

Colin and I went up to collect the children on Saturday (to minimise the risk of me having another and maybe bigger accident), and Rita made a huge roast dinner, which I ate voraciously. She packed up all the leftovers and made up a little parcel for me to take back, worrying that maybe I had got lazy in her absence and wasn't eating properly. On the contrary, I found I had the appetite of three, and the weight was beginning to go back on again as I munched my way through many small but frequent meals during the day. It staved off the nauseous feeling and metallic taste in my mouth.

Monday 1st May

Monday was a Bank Holiday, so the four of us went out for a very nice pub lunch with my mother and my grandparents. Grandad was still going strong at ninety-four years of age, and still driving. Granny was eighty-nine, and neither of them looked a day over seventy-five. Both were clearly very upset that I had breast cancer but over the course of lunch, they realised that I was not giving into the illness or the treatment but facing it head on. It was obviously difficult to discuss any of it at the table with the children, so Granny waited until we had all gone back to theirs for tea before quizzing me.

'I must say, Joanna, you look surprisingly well. A bit tired, a bit pale – but nothing like I was expecting. You're such a brave girl, and always have been,' Granny said, her eyes moistening.

I smiled, and squeezed her arm. 'There's nothing else for it,' I said. 'The medical world has given me a good prognosis; I have a great oncologist who, incidentally, is also a research scientist; and I'm sure that through her I'll always get the best treatment.'

'That's such a reassurance.'

'Also, they found it early and even if it *is* going to get me, it could be another fifteen years off yet. It's not going to get me tomorrow, and I'm not incapacitated by either the illness or the treatment.'

'Are you managing with the chemotherapy?' Granny asked, hardly able to believe, even now, that her granddaughter was on such a severe treatment.

'Yes, I am actually,' I looked faintly surprised. 'I sleep a lot, and have to take it easy, but all in all, it's not nearly as bad as I thought it was going to be. I thought I was going to feel like death for the first week, just throwing up everywhere and having my insides ripped out. But it's nothing like that. I just feel faintly sick – kind of like morning sickness actually – and very drained. In fact, very like morning sickness.'

Granny looked at me. 'But you're not, are you?'

'Impossible!' I said honestly. Granny laughed.

'I'm sure Colin is such an amazing support to you,' said Granny, who had always been very fond of Colin.

'Yes, he is. I probably don't realise how much, actually,' I admitted. 'You get so wrapped up in everything that's happening to you that you stop seeing what other people are doing to ease your burden.'

I loved spending days *en famille*, and we drove back home that evening happily, all singing along with the children's PlayDays tape in the cassette deck, each trying to out-sing the others.

2nd – 3rd May: Mum's birthday

The children were back at school the next day, and on the Wednesday I went for my mother's birthday dinner (Happy Birthday Mum and thanks for all your help!!) over at my aunt Viv's house, which was another enjoyable family evening. My uncle Richard was about to retire, having spent 20 years at O&M Advertising agency. He was looking forward to it, but wondered what he was going to be doing to keep him occupied, having worked so full on for so many years. Although they had already asked him to consult on a part-time basis.

'Just make sure you take at least 3 months off before you start doing any work again.' I advised, knowing how tough I was finding it to let go of work - and I had been in the workforce for less time than Richard. In the way home, I remembered my conversation with Granny about support, and realised how lucky I was to have a large, caring family and so many good friends, who all demonstrated their concern and their willingness to help. I couldn't imagine having to face this without such a support network. While you may not directly notice it when you have it, you certainly would notice it if you didn't.

Friday 5th May

The week trickled past, and on Friday I was back at the doctor's having my weekly blood test. I went back home, and found myself pacing from room to room, restless. Much as I was enjoying this rare opportunity for idleness and relaxation, it was also driving me up the wall. The days had no structure to them, and it was always six in the evening before I had even thought about going out and doing something, achieving something. In my boredom, I contacted work and volunteered to continue with the margin management and job tracking system. After looking at three alternative systems, the board had selected one and I was starting work with the designer/programmer selected. My domestic paperwork was beginning to backlog, although I really didn't have any excuse now. After all, I had all day, every day rather than my usual overdue slog through all the bills, correspondence and school paperwork – invariably at midnight. But now I had time on my hands, I found myself prevaricating – something I'd never done before – always thinking that I'd find my cheque book later, or find a pen later, or go to the shop to get the stamps later. Whatever, I'd find an excuse, and suddenly I was getting red phone bills, and reminder letters about previously sent correspondence. I needed structure to my day, a pattern to my week, rather than just the haze in between that three-weekly blot on the landscape.

The chemotherapy wasn't the only blot on the landscape. The landscape of my bath was seriously blotted again with a huge hair fall-out at the end of week two between chemotherapies – just like last time round. It turned my stomach to see the surface of the water thick with my hair, and when I stood up it all stuck to me. I had to then put the shower hose onto the bath taps and wash myself down! Fortunately I had taken my friend, Celia's advice about getting a bath plug strainer to make it easier to dispose of the hair afterwards. And I hardly dared look in the mirror to see what the fall-out had done to my scalp.

I dried my hair carefully, brushing it gently into place – still ending up with a hairbrush full of hairs – before leaving it to dry naturally. They recommended avoiding the hair-drier, but if I had to use it, to only use it on a cool setting. I was following their advice to the letter. Once it was dry, I examined my head closely in the mirror. Certainly my hair was much, much thinner than the thick batch of hair I was used to styling, and pushing over my shoulder, or twisting up behind my head. But there was no definite bald patch yet. There was still an even cover of hair over my head, and certainly no need for wigs or hats yet, I was relieved to notice.

But my face was looking grey, with huge shadows under my eyes. I looked at myself in the mirror and decided I should have another facial – in fact, I decided, I would book a facial prior to every session of chemotherapy. It was also a relaxing way to spend the day beforehand as I always got so tense and nervous by then. Thoughts of the ice-cap and the needles rose up in my mind, and I had to keep pushing them away.

'Much as there's an awful lot happening in my life at the moment that I don't like,' I admitted to Colin, 'there's also a lot else that I'm quite enjoying.'

'Like what?' he asked.

'Like spending time with the children, playing games or just talking to them, listening to them read or whatever, and having lunches and dinners with family and friends – stuff I never used to make time for – and having facials, going shopping… all that sort of thing.'

Colin nodded. 'I've been telling you for years that it's not a crime to slow down long enough to enjoy yourself.'

'Yes, well, now that I have, I may not ever get back up to full speed again.'

'Good. See to it that you don't. It was completely unnecessary.'

> ## Lesson learned:
> ### It's not a crime to relax and make time for yourself and your loved ones.

Tuesday 9th May

I also contacted the girl from Argentiére that Kate had mentioned, Sarah Poulter. She lived part-time in Battersea, and came to Kingston occasionally so we arranged to meet up for a coffee.

Once settled in the Muffin coffee shop, Sarah told me her story. She'd had breast cancer in 1994. After a lumpectomy and radiotherapy, she'd taken Tamoxifen for the prescribed five years. Within weeks of completing the Tamoxifen, she'd found a couple more lumps. It had obviously stunned her as she'd settled back into work and normal life - never imagining it would come back. She underwent a mastectomy and chemotherapy this time, and was on a different hormone treatment.

I remarked how well she looked, considering she had only finished the chemo six months earlier, and she agreed that she felt well.

'And what about you?' she asked. 'How are you finding it all?'

'Well, I feel confident that I am getting some of the best treatment and advice.' I began.

'I noticed this time round how much more information there was. In 1994, there was *no* information to be found, and what I managed to get from the medical team was scant. I feel much, much more informed and supported now.' Sarah agreed.

'I just wish I knew why I got it though.' I said.

Sarah shrugged . 'Bad luck, I suppose.'

'There must be more than that. Poor diets, bad pollution, stress of work...' I trailed off momentarily, as I thought of work again. 'Do you know, one part of me felt *relieved* when the doctor said there was something wrong with me. I had felt *so* tired for *so* long - and now I had a reason to stop the merry-go-round.' But having got off the merry-go-round, I was a lost soul.

Sarah nodded understandingly, and continued to listen as I babbled on and on about how tired and bewildered I felt, and about the work I was busying myself with.

Two years later, Sarah admitted how surprised she was that I was still so pre-occupied with work and unable to let go even whilst dealing with a serious illness and its challenging treatment. But for the moment, she let me ramble before advising me to investigate complementary therapies. Five years on, Sarah's cancer has returned and she is now battling with the effects of Taxotere – a new drug for secondary cancers.

> *Message for Sarah*
> **Keep up the fight Sarah – you showed me how to be positive and I know you have the strength of will and character to remain positive now.**

Further reading "The world of homeopathy"
on the website www.careerkidsandbreastcancer.com

Chapter Thirteen
Staying positive

Thursday 11ᵗʰ May
The hospital was as busy and chaotic as usual as I made my way up to the eighth floor for my third session of chemotherapy. I promptly had my observations done and was disappointed to notice that I had put on half a stone since the first chemotherapy.

'It's the steroids,' said the young nurse.

I shook my head. 'Uh-huh. It's the food. I've been snacking all day, every day just to get rid of that sickly feeling.'

I was shown into Dr Jones's office next, and she gave me a broad grin. 'Well, haven't you got loads of hair still,' she said cheerily.

'It's feels so thin in comparison to usual,' I subconsciously ran my hands through my hair, then had to surreptitiously dispose of the handful of hairs that came out.

'You're lucky it was so thick to start with. A lot of women don't have such thick hair to begin with, so even with the ice-cap their hair still ends up very thin.'

'If I wasn't having the ice-cap, would I be bald by now?' I asked.

'Yes,' Dr Jones said simply. 'How's it going?'

'Fine, fine. I feel sick for the first week afterwards – but not really badly. Just like morning sickness. I'm eating loads, the whole time,'

'Yes, you've put on some weight since I last saw you.'

I pulled a face. 'I seem to be having such a wide range of reactions. I physically can't manage fizzy drinks, and I've had to empty all the bleach out of my bathrooms as that was really making my stomach heave. What do they put in those toilet cleaners? I've never had such an adverse reaction to a smell before.'

'They put ridiculously strong chemicals and bleach mix into them, which poisons our countryside and our water,' Dr Jones rolled her eyes.

'Yes, well, I'll be buying the organic stuff in future.'

'Well, you're doing very well. How are the injections?'

'Like sharp little pricks, every day for five days,' I joked in reply. 'They make me feel very blotchy for half an hour, and I tend to sleep a lot during that week. But I certainly feel a lot better the following week.'

'Good, they're doing their job then. I must say, you're looking quite well.'

'Everyone's saying that, which surprises me. It must be the fact that I'm not working at the moment.'

'Yes, I'm sure I'd look fantastic if I didn't work,' joked Dr Jones. 'It's the bane of our lives.'

'Well, I'm jolly glad you *do* work,' I said with feeling, but realised what a dreadful responsibility it must be to be a doctor in the field of cancer. It made my own job in brand design seem so selfish and trivial. What an onerous burden it must be to be someone like Dr Jones, I thought, with people like me putting all their faith and future in her hands. I looked at her now with an even greater respect, although she did not seem to be buckling under the burden.

We chatted for a moment longer, then she sent me upstairs to the eleventh floor, to a different room with four beds in it. I was settling myself down for the session when suddenly my mobile phone rang. I'd forgotten to turn it off, and I guiltily rummaged for it in my bag, apologising as its noisy ring invaded the room.

'Hello?' I said quietly and breathlessly.

'It's me,' said Colin. 'I've got a major problem. I have a client wanting to meet up after lunch for a crisis talk. It's their problem, not ours. They need to re-do part of their site urgently, and I won't be able to get to you before about four-thirty.'

'I'll get a taxi,' I said, just wanting to get off the phone. 'Don't worry about it. I've got money on me, I'll just get a taxi home. After all, it's not like we'll be missing out on any scintillating conversation on the way home.'

Colin asked me two further times whether I minded, and I kept repeating that I didn't, so in the end he said he'd see me at home at about five-thirty.

We went through the same process again, the tablets, the cap, the drip, the wooziness. I settled back into it, hating every second of it but forcing myself just to go onto auto-pilot and accept it. This time they put the needle in a vein by the bone of my wrist which made me feel quite faint. Carolyn saw my face whiten.

'Do you want me to stop for a moment?' she asked.

'No, carry on and just ignore me.' I said, putting my head forward slightly and breathing deeply.

Soon the drip was in place and the lerazapan took its effect. I dozed, vaguely aware of an Asian doctor sitting by me administering the chemotherapy drugs. He was much faster than the nurses who had administered it previously, and I said so.

He smiled. 'It's experience,' he said in his gentle, quiet voice. 'I know when to back off, and when I can keep the stream flowing steadily.' I nodded, and decided I liked the fact that it was a lot faster.

Before I knew it, the session was over, which was a huge relief, given its dreadful start. At the end, Carolyn organised a taxi for me. I clambered into the back, staring out of the window. The driver looked at me in his rear vision mirror, and he must have been thinking how awful I looked. *They shouldn't let them out of hospital so soon, whatever her problem is.*

The next thing I knew, I woke up on top of my bed, fully dressed. I couldn't remember coming home, getting to bed or, come to think of it, how much the cab fare was. For all I knew, I'd given the bloke my entire handbag. The thought made me go cold, and I went downstairs as quickly as I could manage.

I found my bag in a crumpled heap by the front door. I opened it and saw my purse immediately. 'Thank God,' I muttered, and opened it. There were still some notes in there, so he hadn't taken everything anyway. I rifled through and found a taxi receipt, marked '£25' and dated with that day's date. I could remember the date of each chemotherapy – not even drugs could eradicate those dates. Obviously the taxi driver had realised I was in a bit of a state, and was doing his level best to prove that he was an honest guy just trying to help out. 'Thank you, whoever you are,' I said, looking upwards.

Colin appeared in the doorway from the conservatory. 'Who are you talking to?' he asked. I told him and he looked at me like I was quite mad.

15*th* – 19*th* May

The next week passed in its usual haze, and I was beginning to get used to the pattern, having set some kind of structure into my day. I had my jabs each morning, then did some of my house paperwork, responded to the frequent e-mails my brothers sent to me, chatted to a few friends on the phone, then I slept in the afternoon for about three hours. Late afternoon I just sat in the sitting room or conservatory, where I could generally chat to the children, play cards or just be with them. Rita bustled around fetching and carrying, preparing dinner and getting the children bathed and ready for bed. All I had to do was chivvy them into bed at 7.30 and read them bedtime stories.

As a full-time working mother, I had frequently felt guilty that I was missing out on precious time with my children, that I would wake up one day and find them eighteen years old and leaving home. Articles in magazines and newspapers also told me that I was missing out by working, and would regret it; that I wasn't investing the necessary time in developing close, bonding relationships that would protect what becomes a fragile relationship during the teenage years. Maybe my children were having problems at school, with friends, with their feelings, whatever, that I was unaware of because I was too busy working, my attention elsewhere. These articles frequently made me work extra hard at paying attention to my kids, listening closely to what they were saying in case there were subtle messages under their complaints that 'Joe pushed me today', or 'Lucy didn't want me to be in her game'.

Over the years, I'd listened closely to what Rita or nannies said about the children, and frequently lay awake at night wondering if Grace's whimpering was just the typical whimpering of a five-year-old girl, or if she was having problems deep down. And were Eliot's spates of frenzied activity perfectly normal for a four-year-old boy, or did he have a food intolerance? (A very popular condition nowadays!)

But I'd always found it so difficult to concentrate on two very demanding roles – career woman and mother. These problems used to whirl round my head, adding to the other problems I faced on a daily basis, and adding to the long list of things I should be doing.

However, this time off work had taught me about more than just nutrition. I found I had time to spend on the children, to sit down and discuss behaviour with them, rather than just shouting at them to stop doing something naughty, and I had time to have long conversations with them about school, about friends.

The most reassuring parental lesson I learned during this time off work was that, despite the increased time investment with my children, I didn't learn anything about them that I hadn't known before. Despite being at work, my motherly antennae had always been fully functioning, and I had instinctively picked up on problems and ill health. You don't need to be the full-time mother at home to know your children, or for your children to know you – you just needed to work a darn sight harder at it if you're juggling a career. It really and truly is the quality of time spent together, not the quantity, that counts.

Together with finding more time for the children, I decided this would be the ideal time to do work on the house and I set about finding builders and decorators to carry out the never-ending list of tasks that needed doing. When I was working full time, I never had the time or energy to organise such ongoing house maintenance.

I also found with my domestic paperwork that the more I did, the more it generated. Reply to one letter, and it opens the floodgates for long-term correspondence and further form filling. How could I possibly ever find the time to go back to work? I wondered.

I gazed idly at the calendar in front of me. Three months had already passed since that dreadful day at Kingston Hospital. Three months, and still – I flicked over the pages of the calendar – another two months of chemotherapy to go, then seven weeks of radiotherapy. I remember thinking what a long treatment it was, but I was now surprised that I was already halfway through the chemo part of it. Only three more sessions.

I looked down at my right arm, which still felt sore from the last chemotherapy, and realised that I had to go through that process three further times. It was quite daunting, but the needles were the worst of it. Feeling a bit nauseous and tired afterwards was nothing in comparison to what it could be.

I was being urged by friends to take up Yoga and/or other meditative forms of relaxation which they all insisted would help me to feel even better. Experience was showing me that the more advice I took, the better I felt so I decided it was time to revisit the Haven Trust which ran excellent sessions.

I rang the Haven Trust and put my name down for the Yoga session on Wednesday, and rang Holmes Place and enquired about Pilates and T'ai Chi. They did indeed run a T'ai Chi class, which I could attend without booking, but Pilates was a course, and there was quite a long waiting list. I added my name to the bottom of the waiting list, and made a note to attend T'ai Chi in a couple of weeks' time. I'd give Yoga a chance first. I felt revitalised and pleased that I had yet another new plan. Positive action.

> *Lesson learned:*
> ***Focus on your health, not your illness.***

Wednesday 24th May

I drove up to the Haven Trust in Fulham on Wednesday – battling through traffic and fighting for a parking space so by the time I arrived, I felt seriously in need of relaxation sessions. They should do this for commuters arriving at work, I thought grimly as I stomped up the staircase to the class.

There were five other women in there all of whom had had breast cancer operations and treatments at some point over the last few years. We smiled politely at each other, while the teacher handed round mats and blankets. After much rustling and organisation, we were each sitting on a mat with the blankets folded beside us, as we were instructed.

'Oh, I'm hot now!' whispered an Asian girl beside me. I smiled at her. 'I'm wearing my wig for the first time, and I never realised how hot they were.'

My eyes widened. 'Wow, I would never have known.'

The girl smiled. 'Thanks. It feels like a beacon on my head…'

The teacher asked for the class's attention and started taking us through the principles of the exercises.

'You must centre your bodies, straighten shoulders and breathe deeply. All movements should be slow and deliberate, stretching fully then releasing. These exercises look easy, but aren't. You'll feel pretty tired by the end of the session, when we'll lie down and relax deeply.'

I watched and followed. Fingers linked, arms stretched forward, above your head, let go and bring one arm round, fingers touching behind your back.

'I haven't got very good use of my right arm since surgery,' said one lady. 'I can't raise it very far.'

'Oh, did you have surgery recently?' asked the teacher in a concerned voice.

'It was two years now, but I never really got full use back,'

'Just take it gently for now. You'll find if you do this regularly it will really help ultimately. Has anyone else had surgery recently?' she asked the class.

I put my hand up, and said I'd had my op nearly three months ago.

'Right, well, don't overdo it. Just do what you can,' the teacher said. I was pleased to then observe that I could do all the exercises, and the teacher commented on it. 'You're doing very well. You obviously exercised your arm after surgery.'

'I did for a while,' I said, relieved that it was clearly already paying off.

The hardest bit of the class was when they rested their legs up along the wall and I had a serious rush of blood to my head that was really uncomfortable, and made my feet get pins and needles really quickly.

'I can't do this much longer,' I said.

'Well, don't push yourself, particularly if this is your first time. Some of these exercises take time to get into. Just lengthen the amount of time you can do it for each session.'

At the end of the lesson, we all lay down on our mats as the teacher crooned in the background about letting toes go heavy, feet go heavy, legs go heavy… I lay there concentrating on letting everything go heavy, but was distracted by how quickly I cooled down, having been really quite hot when doing the exercises. I didn't want to disturb everyone by rustling around with my blanket, but I really was very cold. Finally I tried to surreptitiously open my blanket up and pull it over my legs. One or two eyes opened round the room, so I tried to settle back down quickly.

The teacher continued… *Let your hands go heavy, your arms go heavy, your shoulders*… I quickly let toes, feet, legs and fingers go heavy to try to catch up, but found my mind whirring away and distracting me. Instead I found myself musing what colour the bathroom should be if I painted it, as the yellow was really too dull and boring. Maybe green? That could look nice… *breathe deeply, taking in a long deep breath, holding it then letting go*… And what about the sitting room? That had always been magnolia, but then again with Persian-style carpets, you needed neutral walls… *Breathe in… and… out… in…* I suddenly remembered that I had to change Grace's dental appointment for next week. I'd nearly forgotten all about that… and I had to contact the school about a class trip Eliot was going on. I twitched restlessly, wanting to note things down on my List of Things To Do. Hurry up, I inwardly urged the teacher, otherwise I'll forget.

All around me I could hear gentle breathing. The door was shut, the windows were shut, and suddenly I had the feeling that this was purely an exercise in sharing germs. I found myself not wanting to breathe in deeply, absorbing everybody else's expelled air, so I breathed shallowly, willing the session to come to an end. By now, even the gentle, quiet noise of the waterfall playing on the tape machine started irritating me. I wanted to hear it gush like a tap full open, to feel time passing by, like something was actually happening.

Finally the session ended. I left quickly, smiling politely at the other woman as they all stretched and said how good they felt. 'I'm definitely missing out on something here, but do I mind?' I wondered as I walked back to the car. 'Maybe T'ai Chi will be better for me.'

But I was annoyed that Yoga seemed to reach other people, when it clearly wasn't doing anything for me. When Colin arrived home that evening, he found me sitting in the conservatory flicking through a magazine. From the set of my face, he could see I was in a mood.

'What's up?' he asked mildly.

'Nothing. Why?' I answered crabbily. He nodded, and left the room. I followed him, obviously wanting attention. 'I'm not cooking tonight, so if you feel hungry you'll have to get a take-away.'

'That's fine,' he said, sitting on the sofa. 'What's the matter?'

'Nothing. Everything.' I aimed a small kick at the sofa. 'I'm just fed up.'

'What happened today then?'

'Nothing. Nothing different from any previous day. I sit here. I look at the same four walls. I start little projects, but lack the concentration to see anything through, and lack the energy and interest to do anything.'

'Have you started looking into some hobbies?' Colin asked, afraid of appearing to patronise me. I gave him a look that said I thought he was patronising me.

'I just want this time to be over. I just want it to be this time next year. I can't bear this. The anticipation of the next session, the tedium between each session, the dizziness in my head – I'm beginning to forget things, things I said I'd do yesterday and forgotten today. My mouth feels horrid, all rough and holey.'

'Mmm. Nice,' said Colin.

'And I can't bear the smell of the bathroom. It makes me feel so queasy each time I go in there, which is a lot because I'm drinking so much water.'

'The bathroom? What's wrong with the bathroom?' asked Colin bewildered.

'The bleach makes me heave.'

'Actually, it *is* pretty strong, even for me.' he agreed. 'Change it.'

'Don't give me solutions. I'm just fed up.' I said, still cross.

Colin decided it was safer to keep quiet. With the mood I was in, none of his soothing bromides or typical pragmatism would help matters, so he looked in the papers to see what was on. 'Oh look. The Thomas Crown Affair is on – let's watch that and you can drool over Pierce Brosnan.'

That would definitely cheer me up.

Friday 26*th* May

Amid the general daily activity, the weeks between chemotherapy suddenly disappeared and it would seem like no time at all before I felt that familiar curl of anxiety in my stomach as I consulted my calendar and realised the next chemotherapy was almost upon me. The nurses had told me not to count forward, but I had ignored this advice and pre-marked the three weekly cycle into my calendar. Well, I reasoned, I had children's lives to organise, and the like. I needed to know when to book the children to stay overnight at one of their Grannies. I looked at my calendar, and suddenly realised it was Friday. Damn! I'd forgotten to go for my blood test. I looked at my watch, and realised the surgery was still open. I quickly threw on some shoes, picked up my keys and walked round there, wondering where my brain was. Normally at work I'd have four meetings in a day and would rarely have to consult a diary in order to remember where I had to be at what time. Normally my memory was superb!

'We wondered when you were coming again,' said the young nurse, Liz, half an hour later. All the nurses knew me now, given my very frequent trips to the surgery.

'I forgot, actually,' I laughed.

'Yes, people frequently do forget injections and blood tests.' Liz feigned seriousness.

'Funny that!'

Liz prepared the needles and cotton wool swabs, then prodded the inside of my elbow. 'The vein's getting pretty hard now,' she said, still prodding. 'Can you clench and unclench your fist for me to try to get the vein up.'

I did as I was told. 'It's odd. I've always been told I have good veins.'

'Normally, yes. But the chemotherapy tends to harden them up… that's it. We'll try that.' Liz tightened the tourniquet then I felt the familiar sharp prick as the needle went in. I breathed deeply.

'Oh, it doesn't seem to be working,' Liz muttered, and I could feel the needle being moved around. I breathed deeply as I felt my head spin. 'Sorry. I'll have to start again,' she said, taking the needle out. 'Are you alright? Just put your head down and breathe evenly.'

I obeyed, feeling really quite woozy. 'Maybe I'll come back again on Monday,' I said from between my legs. 'I'm not feeling so good.'

'Let's have another go,' Liz said tentatively, hiding the needles from view.

'Let me get a magazine or something to divert my attention,' I suggested, and Liz disappeared into the Waiting Room, coming back seconds later with Hello! magazine. I took it thankfully and opened it onto any page – ah! the marriage of some semi-known celebrity who'd sold their soul for publicity. I focused my attention on the pictures, and tried to ignore what Liz was doing.

'Okay, that's it!' she said suddenly, pressing the cotton wool ball down. 'Hold your arm out straight and press down hard.'

I took over, and Liz left it for a good few minutes before putting the plaster on.

'Thanks – I think,' I said, preparing to leave.

29th May – 2nd June: Children's Half-term

All my chemotherapy sessions seemed to be coinciding with children's school holidays, so yet again I had to farm my children out to their two very willing and helpful grandmothers. I decided to treat them to a day at Legoland before handing them over and this was a huge success as we went on a day when it wasn't too crowded. We went on the Log Flume, and I bought the picture of them afterwards that really made them laugh – Eliot's glee, Grace's grimace, and me giggling wildly. We panned for gold and got soaking wet, we watched the Three Little Pigs while the kids ate some ridiculously overpriced chicken nuggets and chips, and went on a lot of the toddler rides. Eliot loved the Lego Kingdom and wanted to stay for hours watching the trains run round the tracks; Grace loved the Fairy Grotto.

When we finally left, the children had huge grins, as well as ice-cream, plastered across their faces and their eyes were shining with excitement at their new Lego toys I had bought. At a price, I thought as we drove home, totting up that I'd managed to spend £120 in one day on pure fun and enjoyment. I told myself not to feel guilty about endlessly farming my children out, as they probably didn't see it as being farmed out – and who wanted to be cooped up at home with a mother who wanted to lie on the sofa and sleep the week away?

I've always thought of myself as infallible – I admit now that I expected to find childbirth easy and was sure I wouldn't need an epidural (*Huh!*), in much the same way that I never expected chemotherapy to knock me sideways. But my energy was disappearing as quickly as my hair, and I felt drained. One moment I could be feeling fine, then suddenly I'd barely have enough energy to stand up. But let's get it into perspective – some of the horror stories of throwing up and feeling vile were just that – horror stories. *All* I felt was drained – and as Dr Jones promised me, I wasn't ever sick.

My mother dropped by that evening, on her way up to my older brother James' flat in Putney, and gave me some chocolates, which boosted my flagging morale – and my thickening waistline. She also brought in a pile of vitamins as she had been doing her homework, and found out that I should be pumping myself full of vitamins and minerals during chemotherapy, and after.

A girl from work, Gail, called to ask how the Yoga session had gone. She was disappointed when I said it didn't really work for me and she begged me to give it another go.

"I know I'm evangelical about it, but it really will help you. You're just so active that you have to work that much harder at learning to relax but it is worth it Joanna. Please promise me you'll try again?" she implored me. I promised I would.

Kate had also been on the phone checking how I was, as had Great Granny, and I had switched on the computer to find e-mails from my brothers. All of this helped raise me from my sinking mood, and I went to bed feeling more cheered, telling myself that I could get through this because I had so many people around me that cared.

In bed that night, I read until my eyelids were drooping, then quickly switched off my light, snuggled down and went to go to sleep. This is how I went to sleep every night, and it was a fail-safe method. Tonight, however, as I closed my eyes to let sleep drift over me, I heard my heart pounding away. My eyes snapped open. *Boom, boom, boom, boom!* it went, and I could feel the tension in my shoulders and up my neck.

Remembering Gail's words, I breathed in deeply, held my breath then let go, letting the breath out long and slowly. I did this three times in a row, and physically felt my heart changing pace to adapt to the breathing. My shoulders eased, and my body began to feel heavy.

I turned onto my back, then concentrated on letting my toes go heavy, my feet, my legs, my fingers… and I breathed in slowly and deeply… held it… then breathed out… my arms going heavy… my…

> *Lesson learned:*
> **Yoga works.**

Further reading "The benefits of a positive approach"
on the website www.careerkidsandbreastcancer.com

Chapter Fourteen

Hair today, gone tomorrow

Thursday 1ˢᵗ June

Everything had obviously been going too smoothly for too long. My fourth session of chemotherapy went down as by far and away the worst session up to this point. Firstly I was supposed to be seeing Dr Jones at 9.30am, but it transpired that this was a confusion on someone's part as Dr Jones was out at a conference all day. Then I discovered my chemotherapy had been booked for 12.30, so I now had three hours to kill. I sat on a hard bench down in the ground floor café for two and a half hours before making my way very slowly up to the eleventh floor.

I was back in the same ward as last time, and Carolyn was very apologetic about the mix-up and the fact that they couldn't have 'done' me earlier. I said not to worry, and settled myself in as usual. There was only one other person in the ward, a lady in the cubicle beside me, but she had the curtains pulled around her.

Carolyn said she needed to do a blood test first, which I baulked at.

'I just had a blood test on Friday, which was sent up here and analysed, and Dr Jones said that I was well enough to go ahead with the treatment.'

'Yes, but Dr Jones's not here today, so the senior house registrar is in charge. He needs to check your blood today to be absolutely certain,' Carolyn said gently, seeing me getting worked up.

'But why, if Dr Jones's already seen my blood count from Friday? Why?' I persisted, my voice beginning to break.

'Because he's in charge, and he wants to make absolutely certain that your body can take the drugs. It's for your own protection, Jo.' Carolyn sat down on the bed beside me and stroked my hand. 'Why's it upsetting you?'

'Because it's just needles, needles, needles. I hate blood tests, I hate the needle going in. Once you've done that, then you have the needle for the drip. And we're running out of places on my right arm, and you can't use my left arm because I've had the lymph nodes taken out!' I wailed.

Carolyn suggested putting the canula in and taking the blood through that first, then setting up the drip, so there would only be one needle.

'Can you do that?' I asked, calming down a bit.

'Absolutely. And I'll then nip the test down to the lab, check it with David and we'll be ready to go within half an hour.'

'Okay then. Let's do it.' I put my hand out.

'Firstly, I think I'll give you your tablets,' Carolyn decided, thinking a sedated Joanna might be better at this stage. I took my tablets while Carolyn examined my hand.

'I'm having a bit of difficulty getting a vein,' she said finally. 'What we can do is immerse your arm in hot water, very warm water,' she amended quickly, seeing fear in my eyes, 'for five minutes, then that should bring the veins up.'

So I stood by the sink, with my arm from the elbow down immersed in the warmest water I could stand. After some time, Carolyn took me back over to the bed again and proclaimed it to be ready. I buried my head in my magazine to blot out the stabbing and jabbing around my arm, and finally Carolyn sat back.

'Right, that's that. I'll get your ice-cap… oh! oh damn!' she bit her lip and looked guiltily at me.

'What?'

'I forgot to take any blood,' she admitted.

'Oh? Well, can't you just take it now anyway from there?' I pointed to the canula.

'No. Sorry, but I can't.'

'Oh no!' I wailed again. 'Just tell David that Dr Jones said it's okay to go ahead. She saw my blood test. Isn't it on my notes? Just tell him…'

'I'll just do it very quickly with this little needle, which is much smaller than a canula,' Carolyn said decisively, realising that the longer the discussion went on, the more I was working myself up.

She prepared quickly, but in her rush had to do it twice. I felt near to tears, but fought to keep them back.

After half an hour, I was given the all clear by the senior house registrar to go ahead. The ice-cap was brought in, but I started dithering. Would it be better to not bother with the ice-cap? After all, it just prolonged the whole process.

'It would be a lot faster if I didn't have it, wouldn't it?' I said.

Carolyn stood there, holding the cap. 'It would. It would only be about forty-five minutes.'

'Rather than two hours.'

'But you've got so much hair left. It would be a shame now, because it looks like the cap is going to work for you. It doesn't for everyone.'

'But it's so horrible. It gives me a headache, and I've already got a headache before we even start.'

'I'll get you some paracetamol.'

'But I don't have that much hair left,' I said, feeling my thin scalp.

'Why don't you just start off with it, and if it gets to be too much, we'll just take it off,' suggested Carolyn, and I conceded. As I lay there waiting for the ice cap and the lerazapan to take effect, I mentally tried to readjust myself. I was in a thoroughly bad mood, and it was certainly making the going even harder. I had to snap out of my bad mood, and resign myself to the process. I rested my head back and forced myself to relax. Another girl brought over a bundle of syringes in plastic bags.

'Where's Carolyn?' I asked, not wanting to see yet another new face. Hell, I was feeling shitty enough at it was about this session.

'She's gone up to the other suite.'

'Who are you?' I asked, not wanting to sound rude, but feeling too bad tempered to bother trying too hard at masking my mood.

'I'm a student nurse,' she said and, seeing my look of horror, quickly added, 'I won't be administering the drugs.'

'I will be,' said a quiet Asian voice, appearing round the curtain from the next cubicle along. I was relieved to see it was the same Asian doctor as last time. I nodded in approval and settled back down, finally allowing myself to give into the promise of drugged oblivion that started rolling over me.

When the doctor was ready, he sat down beside me and quietly started administering the drugs. I let myself slide in and out of my sedative-induced sleep, and soon it was over. Colin came as usual to collect me, and Carolyn briefly told him that I had not had such a good session this time.

I walked in through the front door of my house and slung my bag down on the floor, feeling as drained and sicky as all the previous times. Colin followed behind me, wishing he could do something to help, but not only was I feeling ill, I was also in a filthy mood. Best to just leave me be, he decided. He knew if he tried to help, the mood I was in, I would see it as interfering. He watched as I grabbed a bottle of water, and went up to bed again. It was 3.30, and I wondered if I would sleep through again.

In my sleep I could hear ringing. It went on and on with its nagging insistence. I tried to sit up to pick up the phone by my bed, but my body was so heavy. It was as though some force was pinning my down onto the bed, weighing me down. I tried to sit up, to move my arms, even just open my eyelids but I couldn't. The ringing carried on, and I fought to wake up but the pressure wouldn't let me. Finally the ringing stopped, and I felt myself sink back into the depths of sleep again. It was midnight when I woke up again. The room was in darkness, and Colin wasn't there. I crept downstairs and found him lying on the sofa, the remnants of a take-away on the coffee table in front of him.

'Hi,' I said. He looked up.

'How're you feeling?' he asked. I sat down in a chair nearby.

'The usual. I'm going back to bed in a minute. I thought I heard the phone ringing.'

'That was several hours ago,' Colin smiled at my obvious confusion. 'Your mum phoned and left a message while I was out getting that lot,' he said, nodding towards the empty Chinese take-away dishes. The smell was making me feel quite nauseous, and I put my hand up to my nose to block it. Colin saw the movement, and sat up to pack everything away.

'How's work going?' I asked, aware that I had been so self-absorbed recently I hadn't really asked him.

'Slowing down a bit now, fortunately. You can't keep that pace up the whole time,' he replied.

'Are you giving yourself any holiday?' I asked, noticing how tired he looked.

'Funny you should mention that. I have been thinking of holidays… and to prove it, I've got this in my bag.' He stood up and rifled through his bag.

'Centreparcs?' I pulled a face.

'I know it's not our usual thing, but firstly you're advised to stay in England during your treatment, secondly hotels aren't as relaxing as being in a cottage, thirdly if we rented a cottage you would have to cook… so someone recommended Centreparcs.'

'But when can we go? My treatment clashes with every holiday the children have.'

'Take them out of school for a week.'

'They don't like you doing that.'

'These are rather unusual and extenuating circumstances, Jo. Anyway, Grace is in Year 1 and Eliot is in Nursery. How much do you really think they're going to miss for five days? Nothing that'll hold them back academically, that's for sure.'

'So when were you thinking of going?'

'The week after next – neatly sandwiched between your injections next week and your fifth chemotherapy.'

I took the brochure and leafed through it. 'Which park were you thinking of?'

Colin was considering Longleat, and getting an executive villa as they were nearer the facilities.' Seeing my growing interest, he added, 'There are loads of restaurants. We'll just eat out lunch and dinner, and only have breakfast at home. There are playgrounds, games facilities, swimming pools, a nursery… everything.'

'I'll contact the school on Monday and see if they mind,' I said, warming to the idea and certain that the headmistress would happily grant permission. I bent my head to carry on reading the brochure, and in the light Colin noticed how thin my hair was getting.

'When are you going to start wearing wigs or hats?' he asked. I looked up quickly, my hand going to the top of my head.

'What you are saying?' I asked, grinning in spite of myself.

'I'm saying you need to start doing something about your hair,' Colin said honestly. If he couldn't be honest, then who could?

'I don't know what to do with it really. It's getting really very fluffy now, what's left of it. I might go and see Terri-Anne again. At least she'll tidy it up.'

'I'll shave it all off, rather than you wasting money on a haircut. It'll look good.'

'No it won't. I'm steadily gaining weight again, and I don't want to be a bald, fat-faced woman.'

But Colin stuck to his guns. 'Take control of the process and shave it.'

Lesson learned:
**Boost yourself between the 4th and 5th chemo sessions
– take a holiday!**

5th – 9th June

After my injections on Monday, I went back home and settled down to making several phone calls. Firstly, the school said yes, of course the children could have a week off. Then I phoned Centreparcs and booked a villa. It was not peak season, so I had my pick. They even had a gym and beauty centre there, so I booked myself in for a facial and a massage. Then I rang Haven Trust and made an appointment with their beautician there for Wednesday.

On Tuesday, I decided to have a look round Kingston and see what hats were in fashion that summer. I tried on a number of hats, but didn't really like many of them. I wasn't really a hat person. They always felt silly, a bit *de trop* perched on top of my head. The only hats I ever wore were baseball caps, but they have that hole at the back that exposes either the baldness, or very thin hair. Headscarves were bang in fashion, so I bought a couple of those to try on.

On Wednesday, I went up to see the beautician at the Haven Trust who marvelled at the amount of hair I had left.

'We can do loads with this,' she said, which I thought was a slight exaggeration. The woman pulled out a wide array of headscarves in a variety of sizes and colours, and started tying them in different styles, showing me how to do each one, and making recommendations as to what style of clothes I should wear with each.

I had to agree that the woman demonstrated some lovely styles for tying scarves. She chose colours that complemented my colouring and had a good selection of hats that close up I thought actually looked quite nice, though nothing seemed quite *me*. It just wasn't really 'me' to wear hats and scarves. I reluctantly bought a couple, more as a safeguard than a real requirement, then on a whim I decided to go up to Selfridges in Oxford Street. They sold wigs; I remembered that from when I came up to London one Saturday with a friend from school, and we had trawled the length of Oxford Street, ending up in Selfridges and making a perfect menace of ourselves by trying on all the wigs for a giggle. It wouldn't be so much of a giggle now.

The woman in the wig department was very helpful. I explained why I was buying a wig, and that I wanted something that would look like me. I described how my hair had been before I cut it short, and the woman instantly chose a mid-brown, shoulder-length wig with a fringe and put it expertly onto my head. I was suddenly transformed into my former self. I gasped in amazement.

'That's incredible. That is so *me*,' I said. 'Could I try another one? A shorter bob, in a slightly darker brown colour. That also how I've had my hair recently.'

The woman disappeared and came back with another box. I put the wig on I and again, *bang*! I recognised myself. I was beginning to quite enjoy this and decided that, for fun, I would try on a few more. I tried long mid-brown, curly blonde, long black, very short black, wavy red, shoulder length auburn. Finally I decided this poor woman had probably had enough, and that I should stop. I decided to buy the first two wigs, and the woman put them in a bag for me.

'It's odd you know,' she said as she rang up the total. 'My clientele used to be mostly older ladies wanting wigs because their hair was thinning a bit. But I get more and more people coming in here saying that they're having chemotherapy and need a wig.'

'There's loads of it about,' I agreed.

I got home early evening, just as Rita was serving dinner. I walked in with my bags and was about to announce what I'd bought when I decided I'd play a joke – at least it would help the children to find the wigs funny rather than scary. I went into the bathroom and put the first, longer wig on and brushed it into place. I walked into the sitting room and sat down opposite Grace and Eliot.

'Hi,' I said nonchalantly. Eliot looked at me and said hello, and made no further comment. Grace said hello, then smiled. 'How'd you do that?' she asked.

'Do what?'

'Grow your hair so quickly?' Grace carried on smiling in her confusion. Eliot looked back at his mummy, then realised what Grace was talking about. He smiled too.

'I went to the hairdressers this afternoon,' I said. 'Do you like it?'

'Yes. It looks like your old hair,' said Eliot.

I stood up and muttered something about getting a drink, then left the room again in order to put the other wig on. I came back a few minutes later, and sat down again, this time not even saying anything. Grace laughed. 'How did you do that?' she giggled.

'What?'

'It's different again,' Eliot chipped in.

'The hairdresser showed me a couple of different styles,' I said. 'Shall I show you how?'

'Yes,' said Grace. I put my hand on the crown of my head and pulled the wig off. As I did so, Grace and Eliot's eyes nearly popped out of their heads, then they dissolved into fits of laughter as they realised it was a wig.

'Can I try it on?' asked Grace, and they spent the next ten minutes putting the wigs on and laughing at themselves in the mirror as I took some photos.

'I think they've made friends with the Wigs,' I said to Rita in the kitchen afterwards. She laughed as she remembered the expressions on the children's faces. 'I'll try it on Colin later, and see how observant he is.'

'They look very natural,' said Rita. 'And I'm not just saying it. They're very good quality.'

'They weren't cheap,' I said. 'So if you see the children using them for dressing up, remove them quickly.'

Later than evening, Rita and I were watching TV when Colin's bike drew up outside. I leapt up. 'Longer brown or shorter dark?' I asked Rita quickly.

'Longer brown. It's more you.'

I nipped into the bathroom and put the wig on, quickly brushing it into place. Colin knocked at the door, and I went over and opened it. He looked at me and said good evening as he stepped over the threshold. He took his bike helmet off, then looked at me again.

'Very pretty,' he said.

'You noticed then?'

'Yes. Considering when I left this morning your hair was two inches long all over and very thin, and suddenly it's about ten inches long and very abundant,' he said dryly. 'But that mightn't have anything to do with it.'

'What do you think?'

'It's very you.'

When I showed him the other one, Colin looked approvingly at that one too.

'They're both very nice. You need to get the fringes trimmed a bit, though.'

'Yes. I was thinking of asking Terri-Anne. She's coming over to cut Grace's hair in a couple of days.'

Terri-Anne had never been asked to cut a wig before, but was perfectly happy for there to be a first time. After cutting Grace's hair, she turned to me.

'Shall I do a quick tidy up of your real hair, before starting on the wigs?' she offered. I sat down and she trimmed some of the longer, messier bits that were going frizzy. When she'd finished, I put the longer, brown wig on. Terri-Anne put her comb in and went to brush it down the length of the hair, but the whole wig slipped sideways. Both of us dissolved into fits of laughter.

'You'll have to hold the top,' laughed Terri-Anne, as I put my fingers on the crown of my head to hold the wig steady.

'Right. Try again,' I said, pushing down firmly.

Terri-Anne combed lightly through the hair, then snipped away at the ends, trimming the fringe to the right length. 'I'm very nervous,' said Terri-Anne. 'Normally if you make a mistake, you know it'll grow again.'

'That's comforting to know. Last time you cut my hair!' I teased. I put the other wig on, and Terri-Anne snipped and trimmed away at it.

When she'd finished, I laughed. 'I've never had so many haircuts in one sitting!'

'That's a point. I should charge you for three!' Terri-Anne joked.

Over the next week, I experimented with wearing the wigs when I went out. I felt self-conscious when I first stepped out, but then frequently forgot I was wearing one within about fifteen minutes. It was so easy just to sling a wig on at the last second, before I left the house. None of that time-consuming washing, drying and fiddling to get my hair to look good – and it never looked one millionth as good as the wigs, which were quite glamorous looking. Two-year-old Mabel next door was most puzzled. Sometimes she saw me with long hair, and sometimes with short hair, and she would stare at me for ages each time she saw me looking different. I thought it best not to do the hair-removing trick for Mabel – it might have given her nightmares.

Lesson learned:
Use the ice-cap. Wigs are hot & itchy.

Thursday 8th June

Suddenly it was Thursday and I realised I had to pack to go away, as we were leaving for Centreparcs on Friday lunchtime. This was not a task I was looking forward to – it's hell packing for the English summer. But more difficult still was putting the luggage box on the top of the car. This was hard work at the best of times, but I could usually manage it. This time however, we went to lift it up, one on each side of the car, and I nearly collapsed – I had absolutely no strength.

'I can't do it!' I gasped. Colin stood there, foxed as he couldn't do it on his own. 'Let me try once more, but don't get cross if I scratch paint off the car,' I grinned nervously.

'Okay. On the count of three, just up and over, then put it straight down. We'll do it in two hits. First one over. Second one we'll shuffle it along into place. And if you really can't do it, don't push yourself,' he said, then added, 'and I promise not to get cross.'

I used every muscle in my body to get the top box over the car, my knees buckling and the box nearly sliding towards me.

'Put it down,' Colin ordered, holding it tightly on the other side. 'Get your breath, then get it again.'

We struggled for another five minutes until Colin could manage the rest on his own. 'Go and sit down,' he said to me, and I meekly obeyed, which was most unusual. He loaded up the car and soon we were ready to leave.

Sunday 11th June

Considering how awful the summer had been up to early June, we were very lucky with the weather. The sun shone nearly every day and some days were really quite warm. The villa was spacious and clean, and very near the all the activities and facilities. Colin heaved a sigh of relief when he saw it, really glad that it was in good condition and surrounded by trees and countryside. He felt himself visibly relaxing.

Grace unpacked hers and Eliot's things whilst Eliot played with the ducks outside. I got out the literature about the Park, and started deciding what we were going to do when Colin realised how close by some friends of ours were, Gary and Ashley.

'We should ask them over one day,' he suggested. Miranda and Josh were also just up the road, so I suggested they came over one day as well.

We spent the first day fetching the bicycles, cycling around with the children exploring our new environment, stopping off at a huge adventure playground just by our villa which the kids loved, and trying out two of the restaurants. Gary & Ashley came over with their two year old son, William, and newborn baby, Alasdair. After a quick coffee at the villa, we all went to the Dome for lunch, then swimming in the pools afterwards. Gary and Colin took the three older children off swimming while Ash and I sat amongst some tropical vegetation drinking soft drinks and nattering. Colin took Eliot onto the flumes which he thoroughly enjoyed, but Grace declined as she thought they looked too scary. Colin and Gary then dumped all the kids back with us, while they went on the water rapids.

'They're really good fun,' said Colin. 'Can we leave our kids with you while I take Jo down the rapids?'

'Sure,' said Ashley, and Colin bore me off, warning me that it was great fun but exhausting.

We went down, laughing our heads off as we were buffeted around in the swirl, and I said I wanted to go again, so we did. 'This is great,' I said as we set off from the top again.

But twice down the flume exhausted me. 'It *is* really tiring,' I finally admitted, dragging myself out of the pool at the bottom. 'I see what you mean.'

'Shame Eliot's just a bit too young for that,' said Colin, thinking how much he himself would have enjoyed that as a little boy. There were times when he looked at Eliot's toys and wished he could be young again. The toys and theme parks and things just got better and better.

Monday 12th June

On the Monday, we took a leisurely walk down to the bottom of the valley where the Sports Complex was, and had lunch down there while the children played in a huge soft play area between courses, then we had a round of Crazy Golf, and a few games of ping-pong and pool before finally heading back up for dinner at the Pancake House.

On the fourth day Miranda arrived mid-morning with Josh, so Grace, Eliot and I cycled down to the gate to meet them. Colin said to me he that he was perfectly happy just doing his own thing that day, as he thought he might go for a long walk and clear his head for a while. So Miranda and I took the kids down to the Sports Complex for lunch, as this way we could catch up – that is, talk about cancer, chemotherapy and treatment while the children were otherwise diverted.

Miranda admitted later that she couldn't believe the change in me in such a short space of time. I was pale and washed out, my hair was a mess and I seemed rather vague and distracted. As we walked back up the hill from the Sports Complex, Miranda noticed that I fell completely silent, reserving my energy for the long, slow climb up the hillside.

That evening, after the children had finished eating, they wanted to go and play in the Adventure Playground. I had devoured my food hungrily, while Colin and Miranda had taken a more leisurely approach, so I said I would take the children over and they could join me afterwards. After I left, Miranda asked Colin how I really was.

'She seems very "not-there". Is that common?'

'I'm not too sure,' Colin said. 'I can only assume it is, but I think I may call her oncologist and check. I don't think Jo's aware of how vague she is at the moment. She keeps telling me that she's told me something when she hasn't, or can't remember a conversation from the day before, which is so unlike her.'

'I've noticed it from speaking to her on the phone as well. She gets through half a story then drifts off, or can't remember the point of what she was saying.'

Colin nodded. 'I hope I get the old Jo back at the end of all of this,' he said.

> *Lesson learned:*
> *Chemotherapy affects your memory and concentration. But it all comes back later!*

The next morning I had booked a massage, so I set off happily, looking forward to some pampering. I left the children with Colin and cycled down, breathing in the fresh morning air, the scent of the pine trees and the borders along the board walk which mingled together to provide a heady perfume. Everything seemed so crystal sharp, and I knew this would be a memory I would cherish forever.

I found my way to the Therapy Centre and was given a card to fill out. I sat down and had started writing my name and address when I was interrupted by a young woman handing me a key to a locker.

'There are towels and bathrobes in the locker. Get changed into the bathrobe, and wait in the Rest Lounge on the other side of the changing rooms,' the young woman said. I went along the corridor indicated, and did as I was told, whereupon another young woman came and collected me.

'Have you filled in your card?' she asked.

'I was halfway through when I was sent through to change,' I said, handing her the card.

'That's fine. Let me just ask the health questionnaire on the back… Let's see…' The woman started reeling off the questions, ticking the 'NO' box as I answered. I felt a sense of unease, but answered the questions, waiting for one particular question. 'Have you any allergies… eczema… asthma… any heart conditions… have you had surgery lately… are you on medication… have you ever been treated for cancer… have you… Sorry, you have? Oh!'

The 'Oh' was pregnant with meaning and there was a slight pause before the girl straightened her shoulders and fell into a kind of auto-speak, as though relying on a speech that she'd learnt off parrot fashion as some point: 'I'm terribly sorry to inform you that it is the policy of the Centre not to treat people who have had cancer in the last five years as we cannot guarantee that any massages we undertake will not assist in the spread of cancer.' There was a pause, then the girl looked at me, pain in her eyes. 'I'm really terribly sorry,' she added in a gentle voice.

'Don't worry about it.' I felt desperately sorry for the girl who was clearly overwhelmed by the situation. 'Honestly. It was silly of me not to have realised that this might be the case. Don't worry.'

'Would you like to have a swim? Or a sauna? Or maybe just sit in the Relaxation Room and enjoy the ambiance. It's truly lovely. Very peaceful.'

'I'll be fine, don't worry.' I started backing out of the room, wanting just to be gone. I was bitterly disappointed, as well as annoyed with myself for not thinking that this might happen. I got changed back into my clothes and went back up to the villa.

Colin was surprised to see me back so quickly, and by the hunch of my shoulders could tell that I hadn't had a massage.

'I'm not allowed a massage, because of this stupid illness,' I said crossly, throwing my bag on the table. 'It was really embarrassing for the both of us. I felt just as sorry for the girl who had to turn me away as I did for myself. They should write it clearly in the information booklet.'

'Come here and I'll give you a gentle massage,' he said, patting the sofa beside him. I went and sat down beside him, and felt the tears sliding down my face as he rubbed my back.

'It's not fair.' I said. Colin squeezed my shoulders, feeling so upset for me. It was the first time he'd ever heard me say it was unfair. I had been so strong and tough up until now, but it looked like I was finally beginning to crumble.

> *Lesson learned:*
> **Have a note from your doctor if you want a massage.**

The rest of the holiday passed calmly and without any major incident – other than me paying for dinner one night with my credit card and promptly walking out without it. I realised in the middle of the following day and we had to retrace our steps from the day before, hoping that it hadn't just fallen out of my bag. But the restaurant had kept it safe, so I got it back safely. To Colin, it just served as yet another indication that I was slowly losing the plot.

We left on the Friday morning and as we drove out, I looked happily out of the window saying how much I'd enjoyed the holiday. It was ideal given my circumstances – no need to cook; nothing to clean; kid's clubs and activities on hand… everything was so easy.

'I really needed that,' I told Colin. 'I'm so glad you suggested it – I feel so refreshed and more ready to face the next chemotherapy.'

'Only two more to go,' Colin reminded me. 'After the next one on Thursday, there's only one more to go. That's good, isn't it? We're getting there.'

Further reading "Looking good, feeling better"
on the website www.careerkidsandbreastcancer.com

Chapter Fifteen
Alternative choices

Thursday 22nd June

I sat on the train hurtling towards my fifth session of chemotherapy. It seemed like only yesterday that I'd had the fourth, and the three weeks between each one now sped by. It was odd. In the beginning, the three-week interlude seemed interminable – now it was like a couple of days recuperation before I had to be up and ready for the next.

Certainly the injections after each session helped, and everyone I saw said I looked quite well. I felt unable to judge, although the holiday at Centreparcs had definitely revitalised my mental state. I had been beginning to feel quite down with my dwindling energy levels and lack of focus and concentration – and knowing there was still more treatment to come. My hair was so incredibly thin, and some days my eyes looked like huge grey empty sockets set in a round white pasty face. But my ability to judge myself seemed to have gone AWOL, along with my ability to feel any emotion about what was going on at the moment. Maybe it would all make sense next year. But in the meantime, it felt like I'd put my life on hold, and I was merely going through the motions.

Cancer and its many conventional and complementary therapies seemed to take up most of my physical activities and mental ponderings. In the paper that morning there was an article about a woman who'd learned how to be Reiki healer when she found out that her mother had terminal cancer. I had read the article with interest. Her mother's spirits were instantly lifted through the healing and her condition had not worsened in the six months that followed.

I instantly went out and bought a book about healing, which argued that the body cannot get physically well if it is mentally sick. Philosophic arguments throughout the ages had pondered whether the body led the mind, or the mind led the body – but whichever it was, they were both born together and died together, so were inextricably bound up together. If the mind believes cancer will claim the life within six months, it often does. I found this a scary and staggering fact. It was a really powerful example of auto-suggestion. And visualisation techniques worked on the premise that you could make your immune system kill cancer cells, purely by visualising it. It made my head spin in awe.

The more I read, the more I wanted to know and needed to know. Sometimes I felt that I was only going further into the grey mass of the unknown but having read about spiritual healing, I decided I should explore it further.

Lesson learned – an old adage:
The more you learn, the more you realise how much there is to know.

I was completely immersed in my own thoughts as I prepared my bedside table with bottles of water and magazines. Elaine came in and smiled cheerily at me.

'You're still doing well with the hair,' she said.

'Do you think? It feels like a fuzzball, and I'm getting tempted to shave it all off.'

Elaine shook her head. 'No, you don't need to. It's long enough to cover the slightly balding patch where your hair is very thin, but it doesn't show that much. Do you wear any hats or scarves?'

I told her that I couldn't be bothered and people would just have to accept it, although I mentioned the wigs.

'Good for you. You look well. Are you feeling it?'

'I guess so.'

'Guess so?' Elaine questioned.

'I don't really know any more,' I admitted. 'I just know that people keep asking me how I feel, and I just say fine, because it's too complex, long-winded and confusing to describe how I feel. And I'm sure people don't really, really want a detailed description.'

Elaine smiled non-committally. 'Well, we do, when we ask anyway,' she said, as she prepared the trolley. 'It's cold in here, isn't it? I'll get the tub of hot water to warm your veins up slightly. Here, take your tablets in the meantime, and Terese, the assistant, will be in a minute with the ice-cap.'

I dutifully took my tablets, and had just put my arm in the warm tub of water when my ice-cap arrived. This session was proceeding much more smoothly than that last dreadful one. I sat back and let the sedative wash over me, only pausing to avidly read the magazine that was open on my lap when Elaine started prodding around looking for a vein, putting the needle in and fiddling around to check she'd got it in deep enough.

I breathed in deeply and felt my shoulders relax as Elaine stood up to check the drip, announcing that it was fine. Phew! Now I could just blitz out until they turfed me out.

'Hello,' said a familiar voice, sometime later. I opened my eyes and saw Dr Jones standing there.

'Oh hi.'

'Just coming up to check on you. Everything fine?'

I nodded blearily, and Dr Jones smiled. She turned, talked quietly to Elaine then said goodbye and left again. I drifted back off to sleep, awakening every now and again to feel a new ice-cap being put on, then sinking back into my dreamless sleep.

It seemed like no time at all before I felt the drip being removed, and the last ice cap being tugged off my head.

'That was number five,' said Elaine cheerfully.

I looked at her in surprise. 'It was, wasn't it? Wow, I'd completely forgotten that this was the second last one. Hooray! Only one more to go.' I suddenly felt wide awake.

Sunday 25th June

Sunday 25th June was Grace's sixth birthday and she was having a party with another girl in her class, Jessica, whose birthday was the 26th June. A few week's earlier, it had transpired that Grace and another girl in her class, Jessica, had issued party invitations for the same day, same time. So Jessica's father, Chris, and I decided to do a joint party. I'd booked an entertainer while Chris had booked a hall, and Chris had drafted in his family to help with the food preparation. It was a huge success. The entertainer did a disco and magic tricks as the children ate food out of party boxes, and afterwards they all played party games. Parents stood around the back of the room for the last half an hour, drinking wine and munching on the many birthday cakes. I sat at the side, watching Grace's face alive with excitement as she went up to help with a magic trick. I was feeling pretty drained and wasted, but relieved that Grace was having such a great time. Indeed, on Monday everyone at school said what an excellent party it was.

The following week passed in its usual blur of injections, sleep, phone calls to friends and culminating in the blood test. All the nurses baulked at doing my blood tests now, and handed the responsibility over to the most senior nurse, Eileen, who was able to re-angle the needle in order to get the blood flowing.

I had to admit I was now finding the going much harder – not that I ever felt sick. I just couldn't concentrate, felt permanently on edge and rarely felt like talking. Colin seemed to have realised that I was struggling a bit, and I was aware that he was giving me space. However the children hadn't really realised, for which I was privately thankful, and they carried on at their usual pace and noise level. Alice next door was pregnant, expecting her second child, so we whiled away many hours just nattering over cups of coffee and tea – often I would take over my own dandelion coffee or green tea.

On the second weekend after my last session of chemotherapy we all went down to TGI Friday's for an early dinner on Saturday evening. Eliot started to really play up, and Colin had some fairly strong words with him, which left Eliot sitting sulkily in his seat hardly daring to move. Discipline from me had gone out of the window over the last couple of months - I just didn't have the energy to shout. It was easier to ignore.

Saturday 1st July

My brother James' birthday. He was in Hong Kong so I didn't see him, but happy birthday nonetheless. I do always remember even if the thought is not manifested as a birthday card!

Monday 3rd July

I didn't know whether the more 'spiritual healing' side of therapy was for me or not, but I definitely needed some relaxation. I decided I would continue with the Yoga, so I joined a class at Holmes Place. I found it slightly better this time, even the end bit of meditation. I worked hard at shutting out the To Do List clamouring in my mind, and tried to think of warm sandy beaches and waves lapping at the water's edge. I even tried to evoke the smell of pine trees, as I recalled one holiday in southern Portugal and the overwhelming smell of pines had filled my head every time I stepped out of the hotel. It was a much better experience.

The other source of relaxation at that time came in the form of a day at the Sanctuary with my sister-in-law, Anne. For my birthday, Colin's brother Paul and his wife Anne had bought a day at the Sanctuary in Covent Garden. We hadn't managed to agree a day earlier in the year due to my schedule of treatment and Anne starting a new job. Now I was really glad that I hadn't previously used the booking as I really felt in need of some major-league pampering. Anne and I went up there in the train, and had a leisurely day swimming, having 'Jacuzzi's', steam-rooms, facials and nails and lunch. By the end of the day I felt so revitalised - I nearly booked a second booking there and then, but resisted.

Wednesday 5th July

On the Wednesday I went up to the Haven Trust, and talked to a counsellor about finding a Reiki healer. The woman gave me the name of someone, a woman called Freya Browne, and also recommended reflexology as she found this was another great way to help relieve stress. I rang the Reiki healer who advised me that she practised her healing at people's homes. As the children would be out on Thursday morning, I asked Freya if she would have time then. She did, so on Wednesday afternoon I tidied the house and made sure the children put all their toys away before going to bed that night.

On Thursday, Freya turned up promptly. She was an older woman with a very soft, gentle voice… so soft and gentle that I had to strain to hear her sometimes.

'Lovely house. It has a lovely feel to it. Very cosy and comforting,' she said quietly.

'Oh yes. We like it,' I said, feeling like I was bellowing in comparison to this woman.

'Have you ever had healing before?'

'No.'

'And why do you want healing?'

I told her, and Freya made loads of sympathetic, clucking noises as I told her. I felt partly irritated by her, but wanted to give her the benefit of the doubt and accept her as she was. I wanted to see a miracle happen. Could this woman really make me feel different? Feel better? Feel more calmed, and not so restless and irritable?

'Now, what I do normally request is that we sort the finances out beforehand, because often that whole transaction process undermines or undoes all of my hard work,' she smiled. I thought this was probably very wise, and fetched my purse. I handed the money to Freya, who slipped it into her bag, then looked round the room, spotting what she was looking for. 'Ah. That chair, can we bring it into the centre of the room? Great. Now, which way do you like to face when you sit in this room? That wall with the lovely big pictures? That's good. Yes. It's very important to feel comfortable. So sit down there…'

I sat down, and Freya said for me to close my eyes. I did, and she quietly explained that she was going to move her hands around my body without touching me. She was going to find the 'trouble spots' and move the negative energy out, and move positive energy in. I sat with my eyes closed, sometimes feeling like I was swaying. After a while I began to feel immensely tired, and all I wanted to do was sleep, sleep, sleep. I could feel my shoulders slumping slightly, my head nodding and my fingers twitching. Just when I thought I wouldn't be able to keep myself upright for much longer, Freya quietly said she'd finished.

'How do you feel?' she asked.

'Like going to sleep?' I answered, yawning deeply.

'Well, then you must. Just go straight to bed and sleep for as long as you can. It's very important.'

I stood up and yawned again.

'I'll let myself out,' said Freya. 'Go straight to bed.'

I half-heartedly saw Freya to the door, but she was already closing it behind her. Bearing in mind what Freya had said, I went upstairs and put a note on my bedroom door saying I should not be woken up unless the house was on fire, and shut the door firmly.

I slept straight through the whole of Thursday afternoon, Thursday night and woke up at seven o'clock on Friday morning. I couldn't believe I had slept so long. I sat up and stretched. Colin wasn't beside me, and I couldn't remember him already leaving for work. I got up and put on a dressing gown then went downstairs, where I found Colin slumbering on the sofa.

'Hi,' I said, perching on the edge of the sofa beside him.

'Hi. I thought I wouldn't disturb you,' he muttered, opening his eyes.

'I wasn't expecting to sleep quite so long,' I said. 'The note wasn't intended to kick you out of bed for the night.'

'How d'you feel?'

'Fine. Like I've caught up with all the sleep that I missed last year,' I said. 'I feel slightly clearer-headed. Slightly,' I reiterated.

'I'll tell you whether you are or not in a few days time,' Colin said, before getting up. 'I'm just going to go to bed for an hour. Wake me up at eight.'

I wasn't too sure whether the Reiki healing had anything to do with my long sleep, I could only assume it did as the two happened consecutively. But whichever, I felt better in an abstract way and felt more able to cope with the last week before the next session of chemotherapy which was already looming. I suddenly realised that I had been feeling so vile, so bad-tempered, tired and drained that I would have really limped through that last week. My brain had been feeling so foggy that I was barely able to read. As it was, the sleep cleared my mind a bit so that I could at least read my way through that last week.

On the weekend, we were driving up to Norfolk to stay with a close friend of mine, Toddy, and her husband Charles. He's a major in the army, and they had moved from Germany to England just a couple of months earlier. Toddy and I had spoken loads on the phone, but hadn't managed to see each other since she'd come back to England, so I was really looking forward to seeing her again – particularly as she'd had a baby in January whom I hadn't seen yet.

We left late afternoon on the Friday, picking up Colin from his office in Battersea en route, then crawled through London and out the other side with everyone else going north for the weekend.

The last time we had gone to visit them at their previous house, before they were posted out to Germany, it was Toddy's and my birthday weekend (Toddy's birthday being two days before mine). I had decided to bake a cake and write Happy Birthday Toddy and Jodie (her nickname for me). I stored the cake, carefully covered in cling film, in the foot well of the passenger seat for the journey, and carefully avoided knocking it with my feet for the whole journey down to Exeter. As we arrived at their house and I got out of the car, I put my great hoofing foot slap bang onto it and squashed the whole right-hand side of the cake so it read 'Happy Birth Tod and Jod'. Toddy thought it was hilariously funny, and between us all we scoffed the rest of the cake.

This time, I took wine.

We arrived at about nine, and after putting the children to bed quietly so as not to disturb baby James, we sat down for a late meal. Tods and I nattered nineteen to the dozen, to try and quickly catch up before turning in for the night. It was then I realised that while I had carefully packed for the children, I had brought barely anything for myself. I seemed to have packed myself a bag with a pair of trousers, t-shirt, a cardigan and both my wigs – but no knickers, no wash bag, no make-up. I went downstairs in a borrowed dressing gown on Saturday morning and told Toddy my error. She laughed, as Toddy has a very broad sense of humour and lots of things make her laugh, and we went upstairs. She had fortunately been shopping recently, and had some brand new M&S knickers in a bag, and a still-boxed toothbrush. I took them gratefully, and went to get dressed. Colin, when I told him, was not the least surprised and he explained to Toddy and Charles that I was extremely forgetful at the moment.

The weekend passed calmly, the endless round of eating and drinking that seems to accompany young children being interspersed with the occasional walk round to the playground. James was a bright-eyed six-month-old, and he chirpily watched Grace and Eliot running around, dangling toys in front of him and pushing toys into his chubby little hands. Charles and Colin took Grace and Eliot up to see the tanks, which they were amazed at, while Toddy and I started on the Saturday Telegraph crossword. By the time the others returned, we had all of Toddy's and Charles' reference books spread out over the dining table and we were trying to solve 21 down 'Author of Moby Dick'. Sounds easy, but while the book is so well-known, none of us seemed to know the author. Colin and Charles drew a blank, even after I read out the letters, 'H blank blank M blank N, next word M blank L V blank blank L blank.' We all racked our brains, wrote it out, looked up more reference books and each made wild guesses as to what names those letters could be made into.

'It sounds like Herman Melville or something,' I said, squinting at the letters I had written down and trying to fill in the blanks phonetically.

'Oh yes, that famous person Herman Melville,' said Colin sarcastically. Finally I rang a close family friend, Mike Fanya, who was also a teacher and fount of much general knowledge. I explained the reason for the unusual phone call, which didn't seem to surprise him at all.

'Author of Moby Dick is Herman Melville,' he said when I read out the clue.

'Oh!' I said, turning to everyone in the room. 'It *is* Herman Melville!'

Everyone laughed, and I thanked Mike. 'Who'd have thought? That famous Herman Melville. Huh!'

Between us, we nearly finished the crossword – leaving a few impossible mathematical-type questions – then sat down to a lovely Sunday lunch, followed by a walk. It was the beginning of July, but really chilly outside so of course I had to borrow a jacket. The children ran around, getting themselves exhausted before the long drive home later that day.

Once again, I felt more refreshed and revitalised, having gone away for the weekend. I felt positive and upbeat despite my tiredness, and ready to face the next, and final, session of chemotherapy.

> *Lesson learned:*
> **Get away and forget about it all!**

Further reading "Choices in healing"
on the website www.careerkidsandbreastcancer.com

Chapter Sixteen
Tackling the hormones

Thursday 13th July

It was with a sense of surprise that I woke up on the Thursday morning and realised that today was my last chemotherapy session, a fact which Dr Jones cheerily reminded me about as I arrived at the hospital.

'Last one!' announced Dr Jones smiling as I sat down opposite her. 'Relieved?'

'I guess so. I mean, I am, but I'm surprised that it's come round to the last session already,' I said, realising that I was indeed feeling relieved. 'I think I've stopped feeling anything for so long, that even relief is difficult to recognise.'

Dr Jones laughed in sympathy.

'It's a bit scary, as the treatment acts as a type of crutch. You feel that whilst you're getting the treatment, the cancer doesn't have a chance to come back.'

'I know what you're saying, but these drugs are pretty powerful and were only acting as a 'just-in-case' in the beginning. So don't fret yourself into a state. You'll be fine,' she said reassuringly.

'What happens next?' I asked.

'Well, I give you these today,' said Dr Jones, producing three small boxes. 'Tamoxifen. That's three months supply and you take one a day for the next five years.'

I picked up the boxes tentatively and looked at them closely. Five whole years. 'Any side-effects?'

'If you read the literature inside you'll find out it gives you everything… but in reality, the side effects are outweighed by the benefits. Some people lose weight, some gain it; some people's periods stop, some don't; sometimes hot flushes; and in a very, very few cases, sometimes cancer of the uterus – but don't be put off by that as it really is extremely rare. I'm only mentioning it because it's in the literature, but we will be scanning you regularly and will pick up any changes in the lining of your womb.' Dr Jones said the latter part sternly, making sure that I didn't go home panicking about the possibility of getting cancer of the uterus.

Dr Jones checked me over, looked at the Observations Notes made by the nurses, and then sent me upstairs to the Chemotherapy Suite. I walked in and was shown the bed in the far corner where Carolyn was ready to start immediately. She sat down and started fingering the protruding veins on my arm. I winced, and felt bile rising in my throat. I was *so* sick of this process.

'So, have you got any plans for the summer?' she asked chattily. My eyes filled up with tears, and I tried to talk but couldn't. Carolyn looked up, wondering at the silence. 'What's the matter?'

'I don't know,' I said in a strangled voice. 'I just want to cry… and cry… and cry… and just never stop,' I said, burying my face in my hands. 'I don't want any more needles. I don't want another chemotherapy. I just don't *want* it! It's like when I was giving birth to Eliot. It was so painful and impossible at the very end. All I wanted to do was just get up and walk away… to make the pushing someone else's problem… just not be *there*… but I can't. I know I can't just walk away. I know that only I can do this but I really don't want to. I HAVE HAD ENOUGH!' I shouted.

'You've been really good so far, and really brave. I can't imagine what it must be like, and the only way I get through administering it is by knowing that I'm helping you,' Carolyn said, stroking my hand. I nodded, thinking what sound thoughts those were, and I tried to stop crying but couldn't. Carolyn let me cry it out for a while, and just carried on stroking my hand. I was so fed up – fed up with the needles, the sick feeling, the ice-cap and the headaches.

'I don't want that stupid ice-cap. I just want to get through this as quickly as possible,' I said finally, between gritted teeth.

'I completely understand, and if that's what you want, then that's what you'll have. Now, why don't I leave you for a bit to calm down, then I'll come back and set up the drip?' Carolyn suggested.

'No, I'd rather just get going actually.' I blew my nose and looked up, a look of determination on my face.

Carolyn looked at my arm, but it had been out of the warm water for too long and the veins had disappeared again. Damn! 'We'll just have to put your arm back in the water again,' she said, refilling it with hot water and putting it down beside me, as a good idea struck her. 'And why don't you have your sedatives?'

'Can I have two of them today?'

Carolyn wavered. Two really did knock me out, but maybe that was a good thing this time. 'Okay,' she agreed, and went off to get them.

I barely noticed the rest of the session after taking my two sedatives. I slept deeply throughout the whole process, and had to be shaken awake at the end. Colin had arrived before two o'clock, just as Carolyn was in the middle of administering the drugs, and he tried not to watch as Carolyn bent studiously over the syringe – he knew he would feel sickened by it.

The syringes were so huge and the drip kept its regular drip, drip, drip going. Colin watched as Carolyn slowly pushed the syringe down, emptying all those chemicals into my arm. He suddenly felt dizzy and had to look away, but found his eyes drawn back to the syringe. Carolyn picked up the last one in her rubber-gloved hands, making her look spooky. Colin glanced at me, and smiled to himself at how unglamorous I was looking, slumped on the bed with the ice-cap squeezed onto my head, making my eyes distorted and emphasising the frown on my face. My head was at a funny angle, creating some double chins, and I was snoring lightly. He loved his wife more than ever at that moment, and wanted to just gather her up in his arms and tell her everything would be alright. He felt tears jab at the back of his eyes, and breathed in fiercely to push them away.

Finally Carolyn finished, and she beckoned Colin outside. 'Hi, I just thought I'd let you know that she was in quite a state earlier. She was very upset at this session, unlike normal. She's normally taken it in her stride, but this time she said she just wanted to cry and cry. I've given her two sedatives to help her get through this session, but I would urge you to keep an eye on her. If she does seem miserable, speak to Dr Jones - she can put her in touch with a counsellor.'

'Actually, she's been very vague, forgetful and just not her normal self at all. Is that usual?' Colin said.

'I have heard a number of women say this, actually. But their brain power does come back, so don't fret.'

'But it's not unusual?' he pressed.

'No. It's not. Those drugs we're giving her are pretty powerful, so you must expect some pretty powerful reactions, but they won't do any lasting damage,' she said kindly but firmly to alleviate Colin's fears.

They both walked back into the room. 'I'll keep the cap on for another half an hour, so you might as well settle down and read for a while.'

Colin picked up my magazine and flicked through it, his mind more on his wife than any of the articles he was reading. Finally, Carolyn came back and took the cap off, revealing my thin, messy hair. She really does look awful, reflected Colin, but then again, he'd seen her in childbirth as well. Joanna didn't have too many beauty secrets from him.

He woke me up gently, and smiled as my eyes tried to focus on him. 'Oh hi,' I said mistily.

'Hi.'

'How long have you been here?' I muttered, trying to sit up.

'Half an hour, or so,' he said, looking at his watch and realising it was three o'clock already. Damn, his meter ran out in five minutes but he didn't feel he could rush me. We'd leave as soon as I was ready, and just pay the parking ticket if we got one.

The car was forty-five minutes into penalty by the time we got back to it, and further up the road, Colin could see a traffic warden slowly making his way down towards us, inspecting each car as he walked past them. Colin tried to hustle me quickly into the car while trying not to appear to be rushing me. He got in quickly beside me, and pulled out. Another car nipped quickly in behind him. We drove along in the customary silence.

'I don't have to have any more injections,' I said finally. 'None of those daily jabs for my blood count, nor any of those horrid blood tests.'

'That's great.'

'But I start the Tamoxifen in two weeks time.'

'That's great, too,' he said, having read about the amazing success rate they'd had with Tamoxifen curing breast cancer.

Saturday 15th July

I slept, as usual, through Friday to Saturday morning. We were going down to my mother's for celebratory drinks. I slapped on some make-up, a wig and a nice outfit, but still felt that I looked awful.

It was quite a houseful by the time we arrived, as Kate was there with her family, James was over from Hong Kong, my aunt Viv with her family, and my mother's brother Richard with some of his family and my grandparents. Fortunately the weather was nice, at least not raining, so the children all played outside, leaving the house heaving with adults.

'Your hair's looking very good,' said Viv. I smiled, as though sharing a joke. 'What? What have I said?'

'It's a wig.' I grinned.

'Is it? But it looks so you. I would never have guessed, though I was wondering why you hadn't lost any of your hair, because I'd heard it was common with chemotherapy.'

'I have actually got some, but it looks like candy floss round my head.'

'I wouldn't bother what my hair looked like,' said Linda, another aunt. 'You should just go au naturel – my daughter-in-law shaved her head for fun!'

'So what's next?' Viv asked me.

'Peace and quiet for a month before I start radiotherapy.'

'Are you going down to Weymouth with your mother and everyone?'

'Yes, for the last week in July. Colin doesn't think he'll be able to get the week off work, because one of his partners has booked a week off, and Colin's already had one holiday. He figured he'd better let the others have a holiday before he started haggling over time off.'

'That's a shame. But it'll be nice for you to be with your mother, and nice for the children too. I gather Ian's going to be over with his kids?'

'Oh yes. We're looking forward to it,' I agreed.

Suddenly, my niece Isabel was pulling the curtains shut, and everyone looked round to see why it was going dark. My end-of-chemo celebration was doubling up with another celebration – Grandad's ninety-fourth Birthday. Mum produced a wicked, white chocolate-covered birthday cake which the children surrounded avariciously, and little fingers kept creeping out and pulling shards of white chocolate off the side of the cake. I felt my fingers itching to nick a piece as well, but the adult in me managed to restrain myself. I admit, though, that I fell upon it quickly enough when a piece was handed to me. Everyone sang a loud happy birthday to Grandad, then raised a glass of champagne to toast him for reaching the grand old age of ninety-four, and then toasted me for completing Stage 1 of the treatment. Mum cut up the cake and started handing it out.

Grandad started reminiscing about the past, and I listened happily. I was too tired to talk, and Grandad was quite happy just chatting away about his life. I had heard a lot of the stories before, but I listened to them again, nodding in all the appropriate places.

After a while, I decided to go upstairs and have a rest. I felt so tired, and even conversation exhausted me. I lay down on the bed and within seconds, I was fast asleep.

'How has she taken it all?' Linda asked Colin, noticing me sliding off upstairs.

'Staggeringly well. I can't tell you how impressed I am with her attitude and strength,' he said.

'She certainly seems remarkably together from the outside,' agreed Linda.

'But she must get very down at home sometimes?' said Viv.

'Not really – but the children are around a lot of the time, and I think she's trying to mask a lot from them. It's only been in the last few weeks that her normally positive attitude has floundered at all, but they say that's just the effect of the chemotherapy,' Colin said.

'She was telling me she's very forgetful at the moment,' said my mother.

'Can't remember anything from one day to the next, even when you try to jog her memory,' Colin chuckled. 'She gets very frustrated and annoyed by it, and I try to tell her she shouldn't. It'll all come back to her in a few weeks.'

Colin let me sleep for a couple of hours before coming upstairs to find me in one of the guest rooms. He shook me gently, telling me that we were just going to have a cup of tea downstairs, then everyone was leaving. I sat up and stretched.

Downstairs, my mother handed me a cup of tea and I found myself a space on one of the sofas, squeezed between my sister and my cousin Chloe. I felt too tired to talk, and was happy enough to listen to their conversation as they talked across me. *The effects of this are definitely cumulative*, I decided woozily.

Monday 17th July

Our anniversary. Colin and I have been together since 17th July 1989 when we took our first holiday together, and married since 17th July 1993. What a long road we have travelled since our last anniversary!

> *Lesson learned:*
> **We have both helped each other get through this; cancer has only cemented our relationship.**

Thursday 20th July

The chemotherapy was over, but now the radiotherapy stretched out ahead of me. I needed something to lift my flagging spirits, to re-inject my normal positive mental attitude. During the journey home, I pondered the many choices in healing I had first read about, and decided I would see a holistic doctor. Someone called Dr Daniel's came highly recommended. She was formerly the Medical Director of the Bristol Cancer Help Centre, now running

'Healthy Bristol'. I rang them on the Monday and was given an appointment for Thursday afternoon which nicely coincided with my appointment with the radiographer to start planning my radiotherapy treatment.

On Thursday, I took the train up to Harley Street and Colin met me there. The radiographer was an attractive woman called Catherine Piggott who introduced herself as the nicer half of oncology treatment as radiotherapy does not have the same devastating side effects as chemotherapy.

'Basically, in the first week we do the planning by putting Jo under a simulator and projecting laser beams at her. We make loads of marks on her and take X-rays which we then process and analyse. Her involvement will only be about forty-five minutes on the first day, and then she just needs to come back a couple of days later and we double-check our planning. Once we're sure it's right, we then make a couple of permanent marks on Jo's skin, here, here and here, which we use to line the area of radiation each day. They are, in effect, tattoos, only we don't really call them that any more, because tattoos have different connotations.'

'I was going to say, can I have butterflies or doves, or something?' I asked.

'I don't think our artistic skills stretch much beyond a dot, actually,' Catherine joked back. Everyone laughed. 'So once all that's done, then the following week you come back for a ten-minute appointment every single day, Monday to Friday, for six further weeks. Five weeks of that is a more general radiation over the whole area, and the last week is a booster radiation which we beam directly towards the tumour site.'

'What's the difference?' asked Colin.

'Well, with the general radiation, we angle the beam across the breast, first on one side then swivel it one eighty degrees and beam in from the other side and use a different type of radiation. With the booster radiation, we can measure the depth the electrons go to and therefore can aim directly in towards the body, stopping short of the lungs.'

'Do the lungs ever get damaged at all?' asked Colin.

'We do everything we can to minimise any tissue damage in the lung area, but we do need to cover the whole breast area so we do end up skimming across the surface of the lungs. This very rarely causes any damage, so I wouldn't worry about it. However, it's better than we run this risk and make sure we get the whole tumour and surrounding area.'

'Absolutely,' I said with feeling. 'Is any of this going to be painful?'

Catherine told me it might get a bit sore towards the end. 'The skin will be quite pink, and because we'll need to go straight through the nipple area with the booster radiation, you may feel very tender there. But I'll give you some literature which includes information on how to care for your skin while going through the treatment. Follow that, and you should be fine. Honestly, this is not a patch on what Dr Jones has just put you through.' She smiled at her last comment. 'We often joke that Dr Jones's the bad guy and I'm the good guy.'

So once again I found myself signing on the dotted line for further treatment. Surgery down, chemotherapy down, and now part three of the treatment begins.

After the radiotherapy meeting, I went off to meet Dr Daniel, the holistic counsellor. She started off asking me about my diagnosis and treatment, then enquired about my life before diagnosis before going on to explain what they could do for patients.

'Basically, we believe that a holistic approach can help people suffering from cancer,' she explained. 'The states of mind, body and spirit are inherently linked. *Holos* is the Greek word for the whole that is greater than the sum of the parts, and it's by exploring all the parts that we endeavour to make the whole well again. We believe than an individual's self-expertise can be brought to bear in recuperation. The problems can be very core to a state of wellbeing, like losing the point of life, wondering what it's all about, and thinking: why bother? Something might be choking your life-force, or maybe your spirit has become crushed.'

'How do spirits become crushed?' I asked.

'It can sometimes be a destructive view of yourself, which may hark back to childhood – constantly being told you can't do this, you're not capable of doing that, that you always do this… Sometimes it can be a destructive relationship. You battle against it for so long, then one day you stop fighting. You just allow that destruction to wash around you. By identifying this destructive force, and recognising its impact on you, you are halfway to letting go of it.'

'I must say, I don't think that it's necessarily me,' I said. 'I really enjoy life – I can't say I see the point of it, but I really enjoy it. I enjoy my children – I love them to pieces, and I love my husband, and I enjoy spending time with family and friends. I love work, I enjoy the challenges it brings.'

Dr Daniel then quizzed me generally about my lifestyle, work, relationships etc, then explained what she was tapping into by her questions.

'Sometimes we find ourselves living a certain life because it kind of just happened, we sort of fall into a lifestyle. But just because we're living that life, doesn't make it the right life for us. We rarely get a chance to *plan* what we want to do, to truly explore and find our unique purpose in life. What is our life for? What particular things were we intended to do that will deeply satisfy us? Very few people know what their unique purpose is, and even fewer people are carrying it out. The rest of us are just bogged down with earning a crust in whichever way opportunity has presented itself. For some people – like yourself – you exacerbate the demands on your time by the fact that you find it difficult to switch off, to relax and unwind. You're keeping your body and mind up at full pressure the whole time, never giving it a chance to break, to rest and recuperate. This is where the real problems come in, I suspect.'

'But how do you learn to relax? I just can't seem to do it,' I said desperately. 'I really want to, but I just can't.'

'It often takes a while to learn and to blot out the buzz of thoughts, so don't be put off. Some people find transcendental meditation better than other types, because you have to fill your mind with a repeated sound called mantra which gives your mind something to focus on instead of all thoughts and feelings. So you can't get sidetracked by your list-making, or whatever.' Dr Daniel smiled at me, then continued. 'We aim to focus on health, not illness – which I think you do already subconsciously.'

'But I think about cancer the whole time. The *whole* time,' I admitted.

'At the moment, I'm sure you do. These months of treatment seem like a lifetime, but at the end of this year you can put it behind you and get on with your life. Then you must focus on healthy living and fill your life with pastimes that interest you.' She paused. 'Secondly, you must acknowledge the connection between mind, body and spirit, and use this time to treat all three with both conventional and complementary therapies. Thirdly, be an active partner in the management and promotion of your own health – this makes a key difference to recovery. Take a good, long hard look at your life, and chuck out all the negative, self-destructive bad habits, and decide what you want from your life. Fourthly, listen to your inner voice and wisdom. This will guide you. Lastly, redress your nutrition.'

'I know loads about the last,' I said quickly. I was sure if I heard anything more about food, I would rapidly become confused.

'Is anything I've said today making any sense with you?'

'Oh, loads of things! It sounds like you know me better than I know myself. There are certain patterns in my life… which I want to think about for a while…' I trailed off, not wanting to discuss my unformed thoughts.

'People often intuitively know what they need to charge in their life,' said Dr Daniel.

I nodded silently.

'Right,' she said, lifting the tone. 'I have a number of recommendations… I think you probably are doing enough about the food side of things. Are you taking the British Cancer Centre recommended supplements?'

'No. I felt I was taking more than enough with the homeopathy treatment.'

'You should. You really should.' She repeated. 'The supplement dosage has been carefully worked out, and really would help.'

'But why? I've never really believed in vitamin supplements.' I said.

'Because there were cells in your body that started seriously malfunctioning and we are trying to convert them back into proper functioning. High supplements and anti-oxidants help in their way to achieve it.'

I decided it definitely couldn't harm - except my purse. I later found out a monthly supply of the recommended supplement cost me £50 per month.

'But I think that some regular counselling would help you to put your feet back on the ground again. You don't have to decide now, but here are some phone numbers you can contact – but have a think about it first. The other recommendation is learning how to relax and meditate, and like I say, I suggest transcendental meditation as your best bet, to block out intrusive thoughts. There's the name and number of a woman on here in your area who can help you with that.'

I took the sheet of paper that had various numbers on there.

'I think you'd really benefit.' She smiled at my troubled face. 'You've been jolly brave so far. Now, take the time to truly help yourself.'

We said goodbye, and I travelled home lost in thought, wondering if I would bother to get further counselling. Did I really need it? Certainly she had made some interesting observations and comments, but I didn't feel I needed to push this area of exploration. However, as I mulled over all of the comments that Dr Daniel had made, one issue stood out far more than the others.

My unique purpose? If I knew I was going to die in five years time, what would I spend the next five years doing to really fulfil my life, to fulfil that little burning light inside me, that dream? An interesting question – but not one I knew the answer to.

Further reading "Patient's Guide to Tamoxifen"
on the website www.careerkidsandbreastcancer.com

PART III

Chapter Seventeen
Time to chill

I was given a month's reprieve between ending chemotherapy and starting radiotherapy, and in this time I scheduled as many holidays and weekends away as possible. The radiotherapy was due to run right through the summer – typically coinciding with the children's school holidays. This meant that I was unable to leave London for August and September, as radiotherapy is a daily treatment.

I was also due to start the third part of my treatment… Tamoxifen. I woke up on the Friday morning, and sat on the side of my bed as I opened the first box. I popped the little round white tablet out of its blister packaging into the palm of my hand, then stared at it for a while. Funny to think that this little tablet could potentially save my life, and if this cancer ever did come back, the chances were it would not be while I was taking this tablet. What an amazing little pill!

It also represented the next five years of my life. Five years, day in, day out, I would be taking this pill. Today was the first day of the next five years, and there would be a day in five years' time when I would sit on the edge of this bed and think: this is the last day I will be taking this tablet. I smiled at my thoughts at the time because now, five years down the line, I look at the last empty box and am amazed at how quickly this time has gone.

But for now, I had a one month reprieve and I was determined to just holiday. I need to think less about cancer – which had occupied my every waking thought since 18th February – and just focus on anything other than cancer.

The first weekend away was with our friends, Gary and Ashley, down in the country. Gary had organised an opera evening with some opera-singing friends of his in order to primarily have fun, but also to raise funds for the Church.

We arrived down at Gary and Ashley's thatched country cottage late Saturday afternoon. Their house was bathed in late afternoon sunshine, the weather having brightened up as we'd got further and further west. Guessing the evening was going to be fairly smart, I had dressed up and was even wearing one of my wigs, which I hoped wasn't looking too obvious. Gary came outside to greet us. 'This is where the sun is, then?' Colin said to Gary as he climbed out of the car.

'Yoh! Baldy!' said Gary, slapping the top of Colin's head. I looked up quickly, and Gary added, 'Oops! Not talking to you! Your hair looks good – is it a syrup? Anyway – everyone's got more than me nowadays.' Gary smoothed his hand over his completely bald pate. He'd lost all his hair a year ago.

I went into the kitchen, remembering to duck to avoid the low beams. Gary and Ashley had, several years earlier, traded their Chiswick house, hectic London social life and 1968 Lotus Elan for a beautiful end-of-farm-track, thatched cottage in Wiltshire, two Dalmatians, a Jeep and rounded the picture off with two lovely little boys.

'You're lucky having so much garden,' I said wistfully, looking out at my two children running around outside. 'Eliot desperately needs space like that to run around in. He gets no exercise, he loves it when we go to the park – he often plays with other people's dogs.'

'Move to the country. There's a lovely house for sale up the road,' suggested Ashley.

'It's just not viable at the moment. But one day, we might.'

'What's with the Opera evening then?' Colin asked Gary.

'I just thought it would be nice, and the Church needs a new roof so I thought I'd ask some friends of mine down to do an Opera… and that sounds like them arriving,' Gary cocked his head, and outside they could hear the dogs barking.

Suddenly the peace of the sitting room was disturbed as two girls and three men came breezing in, and everyone was kissing each other hello. I had met one of the girls, Carol, on several occasions, and we said hello. I found myself 'air-kissing' as I didn't want to knock my wig off balance.

'You're looking well,' said Carol, unaware of my recent treatment. I just said that I was indeed well. More mugs of tea appeared, and the volume of noise in the room reached deafening levels as everyone talked at the same time.

It transpired in the hub-bub of conversation that there weren't any programmes, and a panic ensued. Colin quickly set up a page format on the computer, while I typed the text in as it was dictated to me, and one by one each of the singer's came over to give me a brief resume of their career for the back page. Gary set it to 'Print', while everyone disappeared to get dressed.

'There's some buffet food on the dining room table, if anyone's hungry,' said Ashley vaguely, disappearing with her crying baby. Colin and I took some food, and I settled Grace, Eliot and William (Ashley's three year old) down on the sofa to eat theirs. Ashley's next door neighbour arrived to babysit, and I gave them my mobile phone number in case of any problems.

'You'll be popular in the Church if that rings,' said Gary, appearing in the doorway belting up his trousers.

'That's true,' I said uncertainly. Colin just shrugged.

'If it's an emergency, it won't matter,' he said dismissively.

'We've only got twenty programmes printed so far,' wailed Dervla, one of the singers.

'We're only expecting about twenty people,' Gary said.

'What time did you say it started?' asked Carol.

'Seven thirty – Christ, that's now.' Gary looked at his watch.

'Don't blaspheme. You're going to Church,' Ashley said, coming down the stairs with a now well-fed and silenced baby.

'It makes no difference in Church or out. God is omnipresent, and knows exactly what I get up to,' he countered.

'Then you're going to hell,' Ashley said knowingly. 'Might as well skip the church now and not bother with the pretence.'

'Not even fundraising will save your soul,' laughed Colin.

The phone rang, and Gary answered it just as Ashley told him to leave it. 'Now he'll be ages.' she moaned, handing baby Alasdair to the baby-sitter. The singers all started trooping out of the door.

'That was the Church. Apparently it's full to the gills, and everyone's waiting for us to arrive!' Gary said, for once looking sheepish. 'Let's run.'

'Full?' yelped Carol. 'But we've only got twenty programmes.'

We all drove up the lane to the Church at the top at full speed in three different cars, and bowled into the church, which was brightly lit for the event. The Church was indeed full, but fortunately the front two pews had been reserved for Gary's party and for the singers. We all filed quietly into our seats, trying to create minimum disturbance. The vicar, a friendly faced, stocky man, stood at the front and made a welcoming speech, introducing the singers briefly. Carol and Alan, a dark-haired tenor, stood up and introduced themselves in more detail, and told the audience briefly what they were going to be singing that night.

'We've got programmes, but only twenty, so I'm afraid you'll have to share,' said Carol, embarrassed by the lack of professionalism, given the huge turn-out. She felt quite overwhelmed.

'It works out to about one programme per pew,' joked Alan. Everyone laughed, as Gary went down the aisle and handed out the programmes from the thin, sorry pile.

They started singing the most well known arias from many different operas, some of which I recognised. I particularly recognised Lakme, which was now known as the British Airways music.

'Makes your hair stand on end, doesn't it?' I whispered to Gary.

'Does it?' he whispered back, showing his bare arm, and we both giggled.

There was wine in the interval, but I was too busy trying to help pass glasses back to the long queue of people to get much myself. Obviously nobody had expected such a huge turnout, but the singing was fantastic and certainly worthy of such an attendance. Gary was applauded at the end for organising it all, and the Vicar rang him the next day to say that they'd raised more money in that one night than they had in the last six months of fundraising. Everyone was so impressed that they had given generously.

Back at the house, everyone made themselves comfy in the sitting room, draped over sofas and floor. Some neighbours of Gary & Ashley's had come back too, and there was quite a crowd. Ashley fed some bowls of crisps into the crowd, and everyone devoured them.

'Shame you can't get pizza delivery round here,' said Ingy, one of the male singers who was from Iceland, a really good-looking guy with suntanned skin and a shock of blonde hair that looked frozen on his head.

'Ashley just told me about your illness,' Carol said. 'I really didn't know. You look so well that I would never have guessed.'

'Sounds like you've had a tough time,' Alan added in his broad Scottish accent.

'Well, you kind of get on with it – amidst the confusion of understand it,' I shrugged, trying to make light of it. I didn't want to bring down the tone of the evening by focussing on cancer.

'Some people wouldn't.' Alan said.

'I felt miserable and incapable when I first found out, but it's been five months now. And I've finished all the chemotherapy,' I added.

'A friend of mine got Aids,' said Paul. 'He was so depressed for weeks. He told me that he wished that if he had to be ill that he could have cancer because at least it was a respectable illness. Aids isn't. It's just an embarrassment.'

'How awful, but I see what you mean.' I nodded as Gary came over and filled our glasses up. I suddenly realised that this was the first time I had really had alcohol in ages. I just couldn't drink it during the chemo treatment.

'I must stop soon. I'm getting very drunk as I haven't alcohol in so long,' I muttered as the room spun round.

The volume of the music went up, more booze was opened, and people started dancing. It's a wonder the children slept through it all, but they were all sleeping peacefully when I finally crawled up to bed at two in the morning.

Everyone was quite hungover on the Sunday morning, and trickled downstairs one by one clutching heads, drinking water and downing a few pain relief tablets. Gary cooked a huge breakfast of bacon, scrambled eggs, toast, mushrooms and grilled tomatoes once everyone was downstairs, while Ashley brewed huge pots of coffee. There wasn't enough space for everyone to sit down in the kitchen, so people wandered outside onto the courtyard with their plates and coffee, and had breakfast in the intermittent sunshine that occasionally broke through the clouds.

'End of July and still no summer,' Dervla squinted upwards.

'At least it's not raining,' said Alan. 'It's the rain that really pisses me off.'

'I agree. I'd rather have a blizzard or a tycoon, than drizzly rain,' agreed Dervla.

'Don't you mean a typhoon?' Alan frowned.

'Actually, I'd rather have the tycoon,' said Carol.

'You're just a gold-digger,' Alan said, lobbing a piece of toast at her but missing, and getting Colin.

'Watch it, or I'll get you for definition of character.' Colin flicked the toast back at him. I sat giggling at the banter, although I really didn't feel capable of joining in. My energy levels still felt very low.

'I think we should go for a walk,' Gary suggested.

'Gary's way of getting out of walking the dogs later,' Ashley murmured with a wink at her husband.

We all busied around, getting walking shoes on and getting the children ready, and finally set off twenty minutes later. Colin came over and walked beside me.

'Alright?' he asked.

'Fine.' I said, smiling up at him. 'Apart from the hangover.'

We went to a pub garden for lunch, and the children all had a great time running around and the sun actually put in an appearance, despite Dervla's moaning about English summers.

'You can't be surprised,' said Colin. 'After all, it is England. The only people here who remember long, hot summers are Jo and Ashley as they're both Australian.'

'Are you?' Alan and Carol exclaimed in surprise.

'I lived in Melbourne since I was baby until I was twelve – and I'm a passport carrying citizen. I've been back a couple of times as I love it there.'

'You don't sound slightest bit Australian!' Alan looked amazed.

'We've been here too long,' I said then added, 'Both my children have Australian citizenship.'

'Yeah. So when they leave home, they do it properly,' Colin joked, and everyone laughed, but privately I couldn't envisage my little babies living on the other side of the world from me. How awful!

Week of 24th July

We got back home to start the new week which was peppered with organisation. Between interviewing nannies for the summer holiday (as Rita wasn't around for the summer), I was also busy with quotes coming in from all the roofers, builders, carpenters, decorators and gardeners during the week and by the end of the week, I felt exhausted and desperately in need of the week in Weymouth that was rapidly approaching.

'It will all be worth it in the end,' Colin said.

'I know. I know. It's just a drag to work through now,' I said scratching my head.

'What are you going to do with your hair?' he asked, looking at the mess it was in.

I sighed. 'I don't know. Every day is a bad hair day. I'm so fed up with it.'

'Come upstairs and I'll shave it now,' he suggested.

'I think I'll give Terri-Anne a call first,' I said quickly, backing off from him. Colin laughed and swept his hand over my head, making the buzzing sound of his clippers.

I went to Terri-Anne's house on the Thursday morning, and she giggled when she saw my hair.

'I'm sorry,' she said, knowing that I was able to laugh at myself, 'but from the back you look like a little old lady.'

I joined in. 'I feel like it too sometimes.'

'What do you want me to do?'

'What *can* you do?' I asked. 'To be honest, if you recommend shaving it, then we shave it. I'm so fed up with it as it is.'

Terri-Anne washed my hair in lukewarm water, massaging the shampoo and conditioner in very gently to minimise the risk of any more hair coming out in my hands. She dried it then started snipping away as we chatted about my illness. Terri-Anne's sister had had breast cancer, so she was fairly well informed about it.

'I ended up styling her hair for her as it got thinner and thinner. As well as plucking her eyebrows, as she always had quite thick eyebrows. With thin hair they looked odd.'

I studied my eyebrows. They were particularly exposed now with my extremely short hair, and needed a bit of styling. 'Will you do mine?' I asked.

'Of course. They could be shaped more, couldn't they?' said Terri-Anne, getting out the mirror to show me what she'd done. 'What do you think?'

I turned my head side to side. It was cropped right to the nape of my neck, and was only about an inch or two long on top. 'It's short, but not as short as clippers would have made it,' I said, trying not to feel bothered by its shortness.

'I've tried to keep as much length as possible, while getting rid of the really frizzy hair that's been wrecked by the drugs,' Terri-Anne explained.

'You've done a great job. I mean, I wouldn't voluntarily have it this short, but considering what you had to work with...' I chuckled.

'When does the new growth start?'

'Straight after the last session of chemo, so two weeks ago. And they reckon it grows at an inch a month, so by Christmas it could be three or four inches long.'

'I'd have it cut a couple of times between now and Christmas,' Terri-Anne advised.

'I certainly am showing a lot of face,' I grimaced. 'I'm used to hiding behind my hair, and now I can't. I feel so unattractive at the moment.'

'Well, you actually look very well. But Bentalls Department Store do Bobbi Brown make-up sessions, and I swear by their make-up.'

'A make-over isn't such a bad idea.' I mused.

'Here, let's do your eyebrows, and then I'll do some make up on you,' Terri-Anne said, wielding her tweezers. She pecked away at my eyebrows, thinning them out slightly and putting more of an arched shape into them while I sat there with a silly grin on my face.

'What's so funny?' asked Terri-Anne.

'I've had some unusual experiences this year, including this… I never thought I would let a friend pluck my eyebrows!' I giggled and Terri-Anne joined in. She carried on pecking away until she'd finished.

'That's a lot better,' she said, standing back to admire her work. 'Get some Bobbi Brown make-up, and then you'll begin to feel good about yourself again.'

Several hours later, I arrived home from my hair cutting and shopping expedition wearing a new face, armed with Bobbi Brown make-up and stud earring, and feeling much more confident at having so much more of my face on display with such a short haircut!

> *Lesson learned:*
> **Have a complete make-over done; it really boosts your confidence.**

29th July – 5th August: Holiday at Moonfleet Manor

Saturday shone bright and sunny, and really quite warm. The summer had started at last – perfect timing, seeing as Grace, Eliot and I were driving down to Moonfleet Manor in Weymouth today for a week's holiday with Mum, Kate and her family, and Ian had come over from Hong Kong with his family. We set off late morning, leaving Colin slumbering peacefully in bed. I kissed him goodbye and promised to call when I arrived late afternoon as I was planning to stop off for lunch en route. The Mum, Kate and Ian contingents were all going straight from a holiday cottage in

Cornwall that they had been at this week, and we were all due to converge in Weymouth early afternoon.

We listened to CD's in the car, and watched the traffic go by. I turned off the M3 onto the A303, deciding to look for a pub restaurant rather than a Little Chef, once we turned off the A303. Unfortunately I shot past the first pub a bit too fast, only having time to catch the words 'Really horrid food served here'. Damn! I'd missed it, and I bet it was ideal as well. There was a car right on my tail, and the roads were too narrow for me to pull over and let him go past. Oh well. Next one.

I slowed down a bit in order to catch the next pub, and sure enough saw the sign 'Great Pub Grub'. I indicated and pulled into the gravel car park in front of the pub.

'Come on then kids,' I said cheerfully, and everyone hopped out. We went inside, and I had to peer through the smoke. Wow! 'Hi,' I said to the barman. 'Where's the restaurant?'

He nodded his head at the tables around the bar.

'Got anything in non-smoking?' I asked hopefully.

'Nope,' he said shortly, pulling a pint for a crusty individual further up the bar. I began to have negative feelings about what the food would even be like. I didn't want the kids in such thick smoke, and I should be avoiding it. I decided to leave without making a fuss.

'Okay,' I said, maintaining a cheerful demeanour. I dragged the children off to the loo before leaving the pub and strapping them back into their seats.

'I thought we were stopping for lunch?' Eliot said, puzzled.

'Not in there we're not. You're too young to smoke,' I said.

'Smoking gives you cancer,' Grace said knowingly. My hands paused, mid-action. 'And cancer kills you,' she continued.

'Ye-es,' I said, straightening up, deciding to nip this dangerous idea in the bud. 'But let's understand something, there are many different types of cancer, and *some* can kill you like lung cancer. Other types of cancer, like breast cancer, are very treatable.'

'Does lung cancer kill you?' asked Eliot, fascinated by death.

I nodded. 'It can do. That's why you shouldn't smoke.'

I shut Grace's door, and climbed into the driver's seat. 'We'll find another place to eat. I don't think the food looked very promising in there anyway,' I said, driving off down the road, my foot sticking on the pedals. I looked down quickly and saw I'd stepped in chewing gum which was now on the accelerator and the brake. I swore under my breath.

'Did you say the 'f' word?' asked Eliot.

'No I did not!' I lied. 'That's a dreadful word, and I will take every last penny from your piggy bank if I hear you say it.'

Eliot and Grace made faces at each other, then giggled.

As it turned out, I took a back road to the hotel which was on the other side of Weymouth, and we arrived there forty-five minutes later – albeit without any lunch. The children weren't bothered as they'd had crisps, apples and drinks in the car. *I needn't have bothered stopping at all at that horrid pub*, I thought crossly as I pulled up by the front door of the hotel.

The rest of my family had arrived already and were sitting on the terrace round the back, while all the children played in the big sandpit and on the climbing frames, swings and slides. I parked my children there while I unloaded the car, with one of the guys from the reception desk giving me a hand. We had a lovely room on the first floor, just at the top of the stairs, with a huge king-size bed and two camp-beds for the children.

'The facilities are great,' said Kate. 'There's a den for the kids to play in, a swimming pool, games centre, skittles alley, board games and a play station, as well as all of this,' she waved her hands happily at the sandpit and playground.

'With any luck we won't see the kids all week,' John joked. Kate gave him a withering look.

But he wasn't far wrong. The four girls – Isabel, Sophia, Grace and Romany – spent nearly all morning in the Den doing activities with the nannies in there, while Eliot and Zach played football out on a makeshift football pitch, using the hammock frames as goals. We lunched each day on the children's terrace, then spent the afternoon in the pool, following by playing in the sandpit and playground before having tea in the children's lounge again. A round of skittles usually rounded up the day to bath and bedtime. Us adults sat around lazily, sometimes taking coffee on the terrace, or sitting in the sunshine. The weather had decided to be really kind to us, and we had warm days, one after the other.

One afternoon after swimming, I had rounded all the children up into a game of football, which dissolved when Eliot decided he wasn't getting the ball enough – and it was his ball – so he ran in, picked it up and ran off.

'It's not fair!' he shouted. 'Nobody was kicking it to me.'

I tried to rationalise with him, to explain that's how the game was played and how once his team got the ball, then they had to stop Zach's team getting the ball. 'Don't they teach you football at school?' I asked him. He shook his head, so I dragged him off to the side, giving Zach the football.

'Let's watch the rules,' I said sitting him down beside me. He watched for a moment as I gave him a running commentary, then he charged back in again to get the ball back.

'I don't want to play this game,' he said crossly, having successfully retrieved his ball.

'Okay. Let's play another,' I said.

'Piggy in the Middle,' giggled Isabel, and Sophia copied.

'Okay. Isabel and Sophia at either end, and everyone else is a Piggy in the middle.' I said, fetching a much smaller, lighter ball from the Games box. The game worked successfully for a while until Grace got annoyed that she never caught the ball, and was always a Piggy in the middle. She stormed out of the middle and sat down on the side, a thunderous look on her face.

'They're deeply competitive,' I muttered to Ian who just laughed. Our entire family is deeply competitive so it's hardly any surprise that our offspring are likewise.

It was just over two weeks since my last chemotherapy, and I was relieved to find I was beginning to feel human again. The disconnected feeling was beginning to dissolve a little bit each day, and I found myself feeling slightly clearer headed.

In the evenings, once the children had gone to bed, we congregated for dinner with our baby listening devices on the table, and I found myself participating in the conversation slightly more each evening. The restaurant was really quite smart and we ate well each evening, invariably having three courses, culminating in coffee and petit- fours, then a port or brandy. We never seemed to leave the restaurant much before ten-thirty or eleven, and only then retiring to the sitting rooms for coffees and liqueurs before finally going to bed around midnight. It was a truly relaxing and enjoyable time.

I often changed into something nice for the evening, and alternated wigs each night just because I could. General consensus on preference was split between the two.

However, the Tamoxifen and its accompanying hot flushes were frustrating, and wearing the wigs in the evening worsened the experience. I'd be sitting there talking one moment, perfectly comfortable, when suddenly I'd get a heat flush, starting from my chest and creeping up my shoulders, neck and face until I felt like I was burning up. I had to peel the layers off so quickly, feeling like I was about to explode, and the wig felt like it was stopping the heat escaping.

'Am I really red?' I asked my mother quietly one evening as we sat at dinner. My mother looked at me and shook her head.

'No. Why?'

'I'm having hot flushes, and I feel like I'm burning.' I admitted.

My mother laughed. 'They're horrid, aren't they?' she agreed.

'Yes. And it looks like I'm the lucky bugger who's going to have two menopauses!' I rolled my eyes.

'You can't take anything for it?' Mum asked.

'No. Not now, and not next time round – my real menopause. They won't put me on HRT.'

'Oh dear.' Mum pulled a face. 'Actually, someone at school was telling me there's a herb that's proving to be very beneficial for menopause symptoms. Red Clover, I believe it was.'

I said I would check with Dr Jones if Red Clover was fine to take with all the other lotions and potions I was being given.

'There are always new treatments coming out, aren't there?' Kate said from the other side of me. 'Does your doctor suggest you start any of these?'

'I have asked about some of them, as the newspapers often write up about new treatments,' I said. 'But she has said that she will let me know which ones are right for me. Apparently there are so many variables even just within breast cancer that not many of them are relevant for everyone.'

'But she will offer you new drugs or treatments if they are appropriate for you?' pressed Kate.

'Yes. She's said she will,' I reassured her. 'I have complete faith that she will.'

On Thursday morning, we decided to go off to Poole to a big leisure complex with swimming pools, flumes, games arcades, bowling, soft play, cinemas and restaurants.

'Might as well do something uncompromisingly commercial,' Ian said, loading his crew into their car. I was taking my two in with John and his two, as John had an MPV.

'And blow a fortune on nothing,' said John.

'My idea of hell,' said Mum, electing to stay back with Kate and baby Cosima.

It was an hour's drive over there, and the children had a bread roll picnic in the car which was just as well, given the inflated prices of the food at the leisure park.

The whole afternoon was a disaster – the rain was coming down in torrents by the time we arrived there. Everyone was drenched just running from the car park to the soft play area. The children played while the adults had Kentucky Fried Chicken from next door, and within half an hour they were bored. Ian went off to get tickets for Chicken Run, and came back with seats for the later showing as the next showing was full.

'Let's go to the pools then,' he suggested.

Everyone agreed, and seven excited children were buckled back into their shoes, led next door to the pools, which cost nearly £50 to get them all in. All the adults winced at the price but dug into their pockets. It was incredibly crowded both in the changing rooms and in the pools. Ian then realised he'd brought swimming costumes but only one towel between the four of them. I gave him one of mine as I'd brought two large towels.

It turned out the pools were all flumes, most of them for children much older and braver than our kids. I left Grace in the baby pool with Mon and Romany (who was only two) while I took Eliot on a couple of flume rides which were both a disaster.

John and I ended up in a pool with all the girls and Eliot half an hour later both gibbering with rage. 'This is hell.' John said through gritted teeth.

'They shouldn't let so many people in at one time. They should cap the numbers,' I agreed. We gave the children another fifteen minutes, by which time even the children were fed up with being pushed around and were all at each other's throats.

Down in the changing rooms, Grace, Eliot and I squeezed into an impossibly small cubicle to get changed, with the kids whingeing at each other. I felt my temper rising. 'The next kid to whinge does *not* see Chicken Run,' I hissed, as we left the changing room.

'I don't think any of us are seeing Chicken Run,' said Ian, coming up behind me, wearing his shirt and a towel round his waist.

I spun round. 'Why not?'

'I've lost my trousers,' he sighed. Eliot giggled.

'Oh no! What are you going to do?'

'Well, after I've cancelled all my credit cards, I'll work out how I'm getting home.'

'Thank heavens I gave you a towel, otherwise you'd be walking out in your pants,' I giggled, and Ian laughed half-heartedly. 'What else was nicked?'

'All the tickets for the film, my wallet with money and credit cards, my mobile phone and my asthma inhaler.'

'Oh dear – pretty much everything,' I said, as he then disappeared into the crowd to speak to the Reception to see if anyone had handed his trousers in. They kindly gave him a pair of swimming shorts that someone had left behind, so Ian then walked round looking incongruous in his expensive suede shirt and a pair of Woolworth's swimming trunks. Fortunately he had the nonchalance to carry it off.

John and I were debating whether it was probably best to knock the trip on the head at this point while Ian talked to the manager of the cinema to try to get him to let us into the showing of Chicken Run without tickets.

'I would if we weren't full. But that showing's full,' he shrugged.

'Then somebody got in on our tickets,' Ian said quickly. 'You stand in the auditorium while I ring my phone.'

The Manager looked dubious.

'We could always phone the police,' I interspersed brightly, and the manager suddenly acquiesced. But it turned up nothing. John and I agreed that we would go home while Ian had to go to Weymouth hospital to get another asthma inhaler. 'What an abortive afternoon. And it cost us something like £120.'

'Like I said in the beginning, we'll blow a fortune on nothing,' said John.

'Did you get your asthma inhaler okay?' I asked Ian later that evening, once the children were all in bed.

'Yes. But the nurse was funny about it,' Mon, Ian's wife, laughed.

'She asked for my permanent address, and I said it was in Hong Kong. She then asked what I was doing in Weymouth, and I said we're on holiday. She said, You've come on *holiday* from *Hong Kong* to *Weymouth*? She couldn't believe it, and I did wonder for a moment what had possessed us.'

'A rare treat to get the family together,' said Mum happily. 'Shame we leave so soon. I've really enjoyed having my family around me for once. It's been a great holiday.'

Colin decided he'd join us for the last night, and caught the train down from Waterloo, or rather the 'Bone-shaker' as it is apparently known to the locals. I collected him from Dorchester Station and we arrived back at the hotel just before lunch. Mum and Kate were round the back, drinking coffee on the terrace and we'd just sat down to join them when John came round the corner looking harassed.

'We're supposed to have checked out an hour ago,' he said. We all looked at him, puzzled, so he repeated himself. 'Last night was our *last* night – we're supposed to be checking out of here this morning.'

'But we had seven nights booked,' Kate started saying hotly. 'It was definitely seven nights.'

'And we've had seven nights.' John replied calmly, and started counting the nights off on his fingers, as everyone else did likewise in their heads. 'Saturday night was one…'

'He's right,' I said, looking guiltily at Colin who had got up at five-thirty to join us for the last night. He looked back at me and rolled his eyes.

'They need us out of our rooms in the next half an hour so they can be cleaned for the next people,' John advised.

'Why don't we stay another night?' I suggested.

'Have they got other rooms?' Kate asked.

'No. I asked already,' John replied shortly. Ian and Mon walked over and in a chorus we told him what was happening. Ian laughed – he has an offbeat sense of humour.

We all disappeared to pack, while Ian spoke to the reception desk to try to find a hotel locally that could take such a large party. They were extremely helpful, and finally located one in Bath that could accommodate us all. We decided to go for it, in the belief that it was only an hour up the road.

Three hours later we arrived at The Bath Priory – a lovely hotel whose management must have wondered why on earth they thought they could accommodate us. The children were very excited at the beautiful pool, pooh-poohed the carefully prepared food and ran wild in the carefully tended gardens. But we had a top-class meal that night once the children were all in bed, and it ended up being a lovely, if unplanned, end to the holiday.

Further reading "Immunotherapy to beat cancer"
on the website www.careerkidsandbreastcancer.com

Chapter Eighteen
Summer radio

The month of August

I was feeling completely refreshed from my week away. The children had been more occupied than they had ever been before, and as a result weren't bickering with each other. The doctors had told me to recuperate from chemotherapy, to get out and enjoy myself – I had and I felt so much better. My feet were finally touching the ground again.

The seven weeks of Radiotherapy stretched across August and September, and seemed to be ages. What did I want to achieve over the next seven weeks – Henrietta, the nanny, was coming tomorrow to look after the children, and she was going to get them doing sports, loads of activities and socialising. To make sure I actually saw the children, and didn't just relinquish everything to the nanny, I had planned an outing each week – Legoland, Chessington World of Adventures, a Star Wars exhibition, a trip to see The Lion King at the theatre in London. It made a nice summer agenda, I told myself proudly as I consulted the calendar.

I travelled up to Harley Street by train and tube, the tube being impossibly airless and humid. The Planning Session was relatively quick and painless. I was put onto two different types of simulators, then they drew complex grids all over my chest and then did three tiny tattoos, one on either side of my chest, and one dead centre between my breasts. I was then requested to come back on Thursday where they could check their X-rays and their planning, and then start the course of radiotherapy treatment on the Monday.

On the way back, I got some passport photos done so I could get a weekly travel pass, and was disappointed to see the pictures. I knew I had short hair, I knew I didn't particularly like it, but one carries around a specific image of oneself in the mind's eye, and these pictures did not resemble that image at all. I threw them in the bin, deciding to wear my wig before getting any more pictures done.

Colin was surprised to see me going off wearing a wig on Thursday, and asked me why. 'Have you got a really good-looking doctor or something there?' he asked, smoothing it down a bit.

'Absolutely. I thought I stood a dog's chance of him fancying me with a wig on, because men love women in wigs, don't they?' I said dryly.

'Nobody can tell when you're wearing a wig,' Colin reassured me.

'I think you can actually…' I paused, staring at my reflection in the mirror. 'I shouldn't have bought the wigs so early on when my hair was really thick. They feel a bit loose and baggy now that my hair is so thin, and it makes them look too big for my face.'

Colin looked at me critically, then shrugged. 'Maybe you can get it tightened?'

'I probably would enquire if I was completely bald, but I wear these so rarely.' And I dismissed the thought.

I left for London, and on the way had some more photos done. They looked slightly better – as much as any pictures from a passport photo booth can look good. I had to surreptitiously then remove my wig in the photo booth, and straighten out my hair underneath, as I knew it would be far too hot and itchy to wear the wig on the tube. I wondered if anyone had been watching, and was wondering at the sudden haircut as I emerged from the photo booth.

The weeks rolled by, with each day taking on a comfortable routine – children playing outside, workmen working inside and I was out for a large part of each day. I left the house at eight, travelling with the commuter traffic up to Harley Street. Ten minutes after walking into the building, I was usually walking out as the treatment was so fast. It seemed ridiculous sometimes that I travelled so far for such a brief treatment – but vital. Some mornings I stayed for a cup of machine-issued cappuccino and read in the library, and one morning a week I had a complementary massage or reflexology session which was really nice. I always floated out of there on those mornings.

I found that I'd felt really energetic at first, and would always walk up the escalators rather than just stand, and two mornings a week I went to the gym on my way back from London, and did some gentle exercise.

'I've been psyching myself up to get healthy again,' I said to the radiologist one morning. 'As of Monday I'm going to start dieting to lose this extra weight I've put on, and I've already started going to the gym and doing a gentle work out.'

'Don't lose any weight though,' the radiologist said.

'That's precisely my aim,' I said.

'No. I'm telling you not to,' the girl smiled. 'Sorry – but if you go changing your shape, we'll have to re-plan all the radiotherapy and start again. You need to stay exactly as you are for the next four weeks. Exercise after that.'

I felt flat as I went home. I'd been really building myself up for getting fit and healthy over the summer, before the long, cold nights drew in and salads got harder to eat as the body craved stodgier food.

As it turned out by the fourth week, I was beginning to feel really quite tired, and some afternoons I surprised myself by taking a nap. By the fifth week of actual radiotherapy treatment, I had stopped going to the gym again, and by the last week I was sleeping for a couple of hours every afternoon. Now when I went up to Harley Street, I'd get on the escalator and hang on to the handrail – not for me walking up energetically.

The outings with the children had all been a huge success, and I had blown a fortune at Legoland with the children coming home armed with loads of new Lego boxes. I was relieved that I'd inadvertently planned for the theme park trips at the beginning of the holiday, and that The Lion King outing coincided with my increasing exhaustion. I slumped in the auditorium, my body shattered, but thoroughly enjoying the fantastic costumes and sets. Grace and Eliot's eyes shone with excitement, and they seemed to be thoroughly enjoying themselves.

At one point, the drums were pounding, the music was ominously loud as Scar was going to kill the Lion King, and as the drum roll stopped, the whole auditorium could hear Eliot pipe up with 'I'm not scared!' as he sat there with his fingers in his ears. Rita, who had accompanied us on this outing, and I caught each other's eyes and we laughed. At the interval, Grace asked to go home.

'It's not finished yet,' I said. 'This is just the interval. We have the other half to go yet.'

'I know,' said Grace, 'but I'm bored with sitting in these seats.'

'They're £35 each – you'll sit in it and get your money's worth,' I muttered and Rita laughed again.

'Let's get some ice-creams,' I suggested, which put a smile back on Grace's face. Five minutes later that smile was wiped off again as Grace knocked over my tub of popcorn and sent it flying, just as the lights went down again. She started wailing. I told her to hush and eat her ice-cream.

Tuesday 5ᵗʰ September

School came upon us suddenly and swiftly. I found myself trailing the children around all the stores to get new uniforms and shoes, which was an aggravating and time-consuming experience in itself. Grace had grown out of everything she'd worn last winter term, and Eliot – well Eliot was starting school. I ignored the pull on my heart strings as I held trousers and shirts against him for size. My baby... in fact, my baby was a huge baby, aged four and wearing clothes made for a five-to-six-year-old.

On Eliot's first morning of school, I dressed Eliot carefully in his smart new uniform and stood back to admire him, and nearly cried. Damn! I was feeling so emotional at the moment. Everything made me cry, or laugh hysterically, or snap bad-temperedly. On one hand I couldn't believe how quickly I had arrived at this point in my life when both children were at full time school. Where did the years go? And on the other hand, seeing Eliot in his uniform served to reiterate how young and vulnerable he was, despite looking grown up and official in his uniform. The children were still so young, barely out of toddler hood, and look at what had happened this year. Look at what cloud was hovering over their house... I pressed my hand to my head to try to stop the thoughts. You must stop this! I told myself.

'Come on kids!' I said putting on a cheerful voice. 'Let's get some photos for posterity.'

'For who?' asked Grace puzzled.

Thursday 7th September

During one of the complementary massage sessions, the therapist had told me about a Nutrition Centre further up Harley Street, which could analyse your metabolic type and tell you what foods you should eat, and what foods you should stay away from. I, feeling really quite overwhelmed now with all the food information I'd read, decided to give it a go as I wanted someone to simplify it for me and tell me what I personally should and shouldn't eat.

I went along to my appointment, having done the prerequisite five-hour fast, and was asked to fill out an extremely long questionnaire which analysed the different systems within the body. Kerry, the nutritionist, analysed all my information, then gave me a diet sheet, which in effect was a vegetarian diet, high in fruit and vegetables, minimum white meat, no salmon, no sugary foods, and no sunflower seeds or lentils, Vitamin A, C or E and a couple of other things. Kerry then analysed my blood over the next hour and a half, and told me the result.

'You have a very high blood sugar – it's 5.3 on the index. The normal range is 3.9 to 5.9, and you were 5.3 when you first came in. That's pretty high, and really you want to cut out all sweet things if you want to minimise your risk of adult-onset diabetes,' she warned me. I saw all the cakes and chocolates I ate sliding out of my reach.

'I can't believe I could get cancer and diabetes all in one year,' I said to Colin that evening. He shook his head. 'The problem is that there's so much contradictory information. The Bristol Cancer Centre say you should have Vitamins A, C and E, yet this woman is saying I shouldn't. I don't really know what to do.'

Colin thought I was overdoing it, making all these changes. 'At what point are you going to stop and just start living your life instead of wondering whether you're living it correctly or not?'

'I just don't know what is enough.' I replied.

'You've made enough changes. You get organic fruit, vegetables, meat and dairy delivered weekly to your door, you're drinking pure juices made from these fruit and vegetables, and steaming what you cook to keep all the nutrients in. You're downing eight supplements a morning, *plus* the Tamoxifen, and you're drinking bottled water at the rate of knots. These changes are enough. You don't need to go further.'

'How do you know?'

'Because, your literature said focus on the health not the illness, and if you take this too far then it means you think you're still ill.'

'Who knows whether I am or not?'

'Then you think you still have cancer?' Colin said, his eyes narrowing.

'Who knows? I keep getting the pain in my breast that I had in the beginning.'

'You're having high dose radiation blasted into your breast, and that's *after* you've had surgery there. I should imagine you are getting some pain,' Colin admonished. 'You have to just recuperate, instead of looking for more and more pots of gold. The treatment you are getting is gold standard, millennium treatment and when there are more answers out there, you can rest assured Dr Jones will let you know. Stop beating yourself up all the time.'

> *Lesson learned:*
> **Stop beating yourself up the whole time; just start living again.**

Friday 8th September

I woke up the next morning to hear Colin downstairs getting the children ready for school. I decided to stay in bed, trying to work out where I was up to. My head felt so full, so full of information: what this meant, what that meant. What did it all mean? I got up and soaked in the bath before going back into the bedroom to get changed. As I reached up to the top shelf in my bedroom for a cardigan, I felt a gnawing pain in my left arm, just on the inside of the elbow. I looked at it, and noticed a lump.

I reeled backwards and gasped. Surely it was just the light! A trick of the light, I thought, quickly smoothing my right hand over the lump. But my hand felt a hard, raised lump. No! No, it couldn't be! I prodded and poked at the lump. What was it? If it moves around, then it's not cancerous. Was that it? Did it move? I prodded and tried to move the lump around, but it stayed resolutely where I'd found it.

No! No! *No!* my mind screamed, and I felt a sick lump in my throat. Downstairs I could hear comfortable morning sounds of life carrying on, Colin asking the children what they wanted for breakfast, the chatter and clatter of normal living. I suddenly felt a hundred miles from it. Totally removed from the happy family sounds downstairs. I was dying of cancer, and soon I would no longer be a part of the happy family group downstairs. They would, after the shock of my death, slowly learn to live without me. And life would carry on. I just wouldn't be a part of it any more.

Suddenly all my fears of this returning, of finding lumps and bumps in different places on my body, all the hopes that this was not intended to be a continuing problem for me… the whole lot washed over me, and I collapsed onto the bed in a little heap and cried like I hadn't cried since the night I'd first found out I had breast cancer. The black hole of an ominous future opened up and swallowed me, fear and pity mingled together, making me cry even harder.

This was how Colin found me when he came upstairs, innocently looking for Grace's school cardigan.

'What's happened?' he asked in horror.

I thrust out my arm. 'I've found another lump,' I whispered furiously. Colin's face hardened before he put out his hand and peered closer. He smoothed his hand over the lump.

'It might not be…'

'But then again it might. Don't you see? This is it now. This is my life. It might, it might not. It might as well bloody be, then at least I'm put out of my agony of not knowing!' I hissed.

'You need to calm down,' Colin said firmly.

'Calm down?! Calm down?!' I shouted.

'Yes, Joanna. Calm down. You'll frighten the children. There is no point getting yourself hysterical until you have something to be hysterical about. Now let's phone Dr Jones immediately, and talk to her. If necessary, we'll drive up to the Royal Free and see her. Where's the number?'

I got the number and handed it to Colin, but he told me to make the call. It would stop me from sitting there panicking. I rang the hospital and got the Senior Registrar in charge of the Oncology ward as Dr Jones wasn't around. I described my lump to him, and he told me not to worry about it. 'Come in during the week and see Dr Jones. I'm sure she'll tell you not to worry – the inside of the elbow is not an obvious site for a new tumour to start, and it would be difficult for it to have started to grow hot on the heels of the chemotherapy you've had,' he said reassuringly. I tried to feel reassured, but couldn't until someone had actually looked at this lump and told me for certain.

'Then we go up to the Royal Free and wait until Dr Jones, or somebody else senior, can see you,' said Colin decisively, mentally scrubbing out all the plans he'd made for his working day. 'Let's drop the kids off at school and go.'

'I'll ring Teresa, Dr Jones's secretary and tell her,' I nodded, relieved that finally there was a plan of action. Teresa explained that Dr Jones was actually out all day, but if I went straight to the Oncology ward, she would ensure somebody saw me.

We arrived at the hospital a couple of hours later. Colin told me to go on up, and that he would meet me upstairs in the Oncology Ward. I went upstairs and was told to wait for a while. Every fifteen or so minutes, somebody would come along with a different request. Some was form-filling, one was a urine sample, one a temperature and blood pressure test, another a blood test.

'You'll find it difficult,' I warned the latter nurse, secretly fuming that I had to have another blood test. I just wanted the lump looked at, not more blood taken!

'Oh? Okay. I'll use the needle then,' said the nurse. 'It'll probably make it easier.'

I didn't bother to enquire why. I no longer wanted answers to questions, other than what was this lump on my arm.

'The senior registrar will be up as soon as possible,' the nurse said, depositing me back on the mock-leather chair.

An hour had passed by the time the senior registrar came up. He sat down beside me in the open corridor, not having a room he could take me into as he was on his rounds.

'Your blood pressure's very low, and your temperatures slightly raised. We think you might be harbouring a small bug in there, so we're going to give you some antibiotics,' he said.

'That's interesting, but that's not why I came here.'

'Oh?' he looked amazed. 'Why did you come here then?'

'I found another lump,' I put my arm out, and the doctor felt the lump.

'I think that's a lymphoma. Nothing to worry about,' he said dismissively. 'It wouldn't be a tumour – they don't go there.'

'Oh, okay.'

'But it's good that you came, because you've probably halted a bug in its early development,' he smiled at me, pleased. 'Take this down to the pharmacy and get them to give you the tablets. Take two immediately.'

He stood up, shook my hand and sped off to sort out the next problem. I joined Colin outside the room.

'So what did they say?' he asked. I told him, feeling slightly sheepish about my earlier hysteria. 'Oh, that's good. So we've lost a lump and gained a bug,' he said. I nodded. 'I think you need to calm down about lumps and bumps on your body, Jo. You've had them before and they've been meaningless, and you'll probably have them again. You need to learn to trust life.'

'Easier said than done,' I muttered.

> *Lesson learned:*
> **REITERATE** *– stop beating yourself up and just start living your life!!!!!*

Further reading "A Patient's Guide to Radiotherapy"
on the website www.careerkidsandbreastcancer.com

Chapter Nineteen
Life after cancer

Thursday 21st September

I realised very quickly that I had felt rather secure during the treatment, and now with the radiotherapy treatment having finished last week, I suddenly felt vulnerable and exposed. My first scan wasn't for months. I didn't have to see any doctors, report to anybody, or have anyone check whether the tumour was coming back. It was, I felt, just up to me. I had to eat properly, look after myself, not get stressed or overtired. Above all, I needed to believe all these things were going to keep the cancer at bay – that and the Tamoxifen, of course.

During my last visit to Dr Jones at the end of September, she had offered me a further hormone treatment – Zolodex.

'You said when you first visited me that you wanted everything – for me to throw the book at you and maximise all your chances?' she said, in a slightly challenging tone. I nodded in agreement. 'Well, Zolodex is a hormone treatment that is ideal for your specific type of cancer, that being an oestrogen and progesterone positive cancer.' She went on to explain that it was still coming out of research trials, but was proving to aid recuperation by inducing a false menopause, thus suppressing the oestrogen and progesterone in the body – again starving any cancerous cells.

'Excellent,' I agreed readily. But Dr Jones seemed hesitant. I nodded again, to urge her on.

'It's administered by injection… into the fatty area around the stomach… once every four weeks… for two years.' Scribbling on a piece of paper, she continued, 'Seeing as you're here, you may as well have the first one now.' She looked up smiling, and indicated where I should sign the form to agree to the treatment.

I paused. An injection? Another injection? Hadn't I had enough of them, could I really handle two more years of injections? And what about the side effects? Do I want anymore treatment, with its resulting lethargy, bloating, indecision, etc?

'What are the side effects?' I asked.

'Menopausal really - hot flushes, night sweats, possible weight gain...'Dr Jones smiled somewhat cynically as she listed the effects. But I knew that Dr Jones told me the truth, that she wasn't holding back and at worst this is what I could expect.

But could I turn down a treatment for cancer? No. Of course not. The real issue was the potential side effect of not taking the treatments offered. I sighed heavily as I signed the piece of paper, before saying goodbye to Dr Jones and heading off downstairs for injection number one out of twenty-six.

I went downstairs into the chemo suite where I was given some topical anaesthetic to rub onto my stomach and a large plaster to stop the cream from rubbing off. I complied with their instructions (and rather stupidly no early warning bells went off regarding the need for anaesthetic!). I waited for my injection, planning to go window shopping along Oxford Street afterwards (as I was in Harley Street). Finally my injection was ready, and I was taken into a surgery.

'Do you want to lie down for this?' the nurse asked me.

'Is that the best angle?' I asked foolishly. The chemotherapy really had done things to my brain. But the shock still registered when I saw the size of the needle. 'What's that?' I asked.

'The Zolodex injection.' The nurse said surprised, quickly checking her notes to see if she had the right patient for the right treatment.

I raised my eyebrows, suddenly understanding why they'd given me a topical anaesthetic, and decided that lying down probably was an excellent position in which to receive this needle. Fortunately, I had a generous amount of fat around my stomach, as I had gained nearly two stone in weight throughout the treatment.

After that, I decided to hell with window shopping. I was going to spend money!

Everybody I met or spoke to on the phone commented how pleased I must be now that the main treatment was finished, but privately I didn't know how I felt. Of course I didn't want the treatment to go on. My breast had started feeling really quite sore after the last radiotherapy booster session, and incredibly itchy. I found myself scooping aqueous cream straight out of the pot in the fridge and rubbing it in, hiding behind the fridge door so the children didn't see me and wonder what on earth I was up to.

But why didn't I feel more elated? Everyone else around me was over the moon for me that my treatment had finished. When I saw my radiologist on the last day of treatment, I mentioned that I was feeling a bit flat.

'You will, probably,' Catherine Piggott said kindly. 'You've been through a lot. Just take things easy, start getting some of your old routine back into your life and by this time next year this will seem a rather bad dream.'

Anyway, I rationalised, the treatment hadn't really finished - not with two years of Zolodex and five years of Tamoxifen.

I realised that I needed to return to reality; I needed to get some distance between this whole unexpected year and what had always previously been normality. It's difficult to get a perspective on life, on recent events and what they mean to you while you are still so in the thick of them. I needed the distraction of work to think about something other than cancer for a while, then I was sure I could look back and maybe understand it all a bit better. Although, even as I thought about it, I didn't know what I was seeking to understand.

Dr Daniel advised that I went back to work part time initially. 'You've been through a lot this year,' she said, 'and whilst you need a lot of time to think about things, you also need to gain perspective. That's best done by trying to return to "normality"...

233

but don't start overloading yourself, or you'll end up in a pickle of a mess.'

Tuesday 26th September

So I rang my boss, Pete, and suggested meeting him for lunch to discuss my return to work.

'Good to see you looking so well,' he said, hugging me. 'You're beginning to look more like your old self again.'

'With considerably less hair,' I said, running my fingers through my cropped cut.

'More than you had last time I saw you,' he joked. Towering over me, he had been easily able to see the balding patches I'd developed at the end of July.

We settled down to eat before I mentioned work. 'I was thinking of coming in one afternoon a week throughout October, then scaling it up to working half a week throughout November and December.'

'Great,' said Pete. 'We'll look forward to having you back.'

'It's then a question of what I'll be doing…' I began.

'We've thought about that. Obviously we don't want to put you in front of clients immediately, so we decided you could write all the new business proposals. You're good at writing, and we need someone to do it. Dave and I just don't have the time.'

'Great,' I smiled. 'How are things going at work?'

Pete launched into the new pitches they had coming up, the new projects won, how busy the designers were, how much income they had coming in, the profitability figures and detailed information that I generally absorbed without even thinking about it. Now I had difficulty trying to understand what he was talking about.

Pete sensed my vagueness and changed tack. 'Here. Have a look at these.' He put some holiday brochures down in front of me. 'I've

234

just booked for me and my wife to go to Tanzania on safari for a week, in a couple of weeks' time.'

I leafed through the brochure enviously. 'Lucky thing,' I said, remembering Dr Daniel's suggestion. On my way back from Kingston later that day I picked up some more brochures - this time venturing slightly further afield - the Caribbean and Indian Ocean - to show Colin that evening. He was all for it, as he desperately needed a break, and we agreed we'd go – just the two of us – during term-time, leaving the children with Rita during the week and my mother at weekends.

'Let's for once in our lives spend some money on ourselves,' I said, pointing out some beautiful and romantic hideaways, white tropical villas on vast stretches of pale sandy beach, palm trees waving gently. I could almost feel the warmth coming off the page, smell the salty, fresh sea air and feel sand under foot.

'Absolutely. Let's stop living life like it's a dress rehearsal, and we're waiting for the first night to start,' Colin agreed. We determined to have a holiday of a lifetime - the honeymoon we'd never had - and set about planning it.

Monday 2nd October

The following week, I started going back to work two days a week. I timed it deliberately to coincide with a weekly catch-up meeting, where everyone discussed what cases they were working on. I sat down at the meeting table, not recognising a couple of faces, and suddenly felt myself like the new girl. How silly, I told myself. You've been here four years, and you're a senior member of staff.

But later that evening I found myself feeling really quite depressed, and realised that it was because of going back into work. Seven months off was a long time, and everyone had juggled around to cover all the things that I usually did. Suddenly other people were filling my role, and I was left feeling redundant and unneeded. I knew it was silly – heavens, it was the fact that other people had been asked to do my job that gave my previous tasks validation. If they'd just dropped them like a hot potato, I'd have wondered did the tasks ever need doing in the first place. And at the end of the day, they were a business and couldn't be held back each time somebody goes off sick – whether it's one day or seven months.

What I was having to acknowledge very quickly was that I had to find a new 'normality'. Things would never be the same as they were before. Events change people. Time moves on and you have to find your new place. Over the next year, this was to prove a far harder and more emotional challenge than the treatment I had just gone through. I so longed for the normality that I had once known, but that had been taken away forever. I could never again be the person that I once was, either in my own eyes or other people's view of me. I had to get with the new programme.

October 2000

The effects of the Zolodex injections provided the next hurdle to overcome. If I'd thought the hot flushes caused by the Tamoxifen were bad, they paled into insignificance beside the hot flushes and sweats I was getting now. I would wake up at two in the morning absolutely drenched, as though I was running a really high fever. During the day, my cardigan and jackets were on and off every half hour and I went from physically shivering in my seat to whipping everything off and languishing spread-eagled, fanning myself with whatever was nearest to hand. Barely tolerable at home, it was uncomfortable and extremely embarrassing at work. Sitting in meetings, I tried to add or remove layers as surreptitiously as possible but there's something about a woman stripping off the layers that draws the eyes of every single male in the room. I would smile back slightly apologetically.

I bought myself a little battery-operated desk fan. Despite the fact that it was mid-winter, I managed to get through a four-pack of batteries per week.

November 2000

Life began to take on a pattern – two days a week in the office, once weekly Yoga sessions, trying to include at least ten minutes of meditation a day, and listening to the children doing their homework after school. Suddenly life seemed quite calm, and I found my head clearing. I was able to think for the first time in months. I looked back on that period of chemotherapy now, and laughed at how I had run around meeting people for lunch, saying I felt fine when really I felt awful – so constantly drained of energy and so disconnected. *Now*, I thought, I feel fine. But not then, definitely not then. But it was probably some defence-mechanism… tell yourself often enough that you're well, and you will be.

'I suppose I do just have to get on with it now, don't I, and trust that the cancer won't come back?' I said to Colin one evening.

'Not every headache or every sore throat is an indication that this has come back,' he said.

'No.' I agreed, then looked at him from under my eyelashes. 'But will you keep reminding me of that? I may forget occasionally.'

'What you also have to realise,' he continued, 'is that any day now, within the next months or maybe years, you'll read an article in the paper saying that there is a new treatment, and that chemotherapy is barbaric and unnecessary. Or radiation causes cancer. Or something… but you just have to put that aside. You've been given the gold standard treatment available *this* year. Next year, it may be different.'

He was right. Treatments would get better year after year, and at least if it came back, I would then get the gold standard treatment for that year. The fact is, Colin reminded me, they were unravelling the human genome really fast now, and chances were that within, say, Grace's lifetime, diseases like cancer would be completely curable, if not avoidable. The answer lay in genomic research, Colin assured me, as he'd had been reading up on it. 'They will find a cure,' he added confidently.

December 2000

We spent a quiet Christmas at home with the children, just enjoying some time together. It had been such a hectic and overwhelming year that we felt exhausted. Neither of us had the energy to even get in the car and drive to see anyone. It was very peaceful, and Colin and I looked forward to seeing the back of the year 2000. We toasted in 2001, both privately requesting a better year. We were certainly aiming to get off to a good start by having our two week Caribbean holiday.

January 2001

The Caribbean proved to be everything promised in the books and brochures. Not only because of the pleasurable impact of heat hitting us in the face as we stepped off the plane - when there was snow on the ground in England- but also because of the comfort and rustic character of the first place we stayed - Young Island, off the coast of St Vincent; and the sheer luxury and fun at the second place we stayed in, The Firefly in Mustique.

We obviously chose well, as the Firefly has since been named as one of the top ten hotels of the world, and we spent a leisurely week on empty, sandy beaches and drinking cocktails at the bar of the Firefly against a setting Caribbean sun. The holiday was over far too quickly, but we vowed to return again.

25th January 2001

I was seeing Dr Jones on a monthly basis for the first six months following completion of chemo and radiotherapy, which I was glad about as I needed constant reassurance that I was alright.

'How are you finding the Zolodex injections?' she asked, pulling a face.

'Oh, they're horrid,' I smiled back. 'But not as horrid as the night sweats and hot flushes, which I find extremely uncomfortable and very embarrassing – particularly in client meetings as I can't even explain to them why I'm sitting in a skimpy outfit beside an open window, glowing like a Belisha beacon, when there's a howling gale outside!'

Dr Jones laughed. 'It subsides,' she said. 'How are you feeling, otherwise?'

'Fine. Fine,' I said, thinking hard. 'My bones ache something chronic, though. I groan like an old woman every time I stand up, and I can actually hear my knees creaking. I don't know what that's about.'

'That'll be the Zolodex too.'

'Really? Why?' I asked, amazed.

'Well, you're having a false menopause, so you're experiencing a sort of ageing process.' She said. I looked suitably horrified. 'Don't worry – it's not the wrinkles and grey hairs sort of ageing. But you must expect some stiff joints, hot flushes…'

'Unable to sleep at night? Waking up ten minutes after I've gone to sleep *every* single night, then being unable to get back to sleep until about two or three hours later?'

'Yes. Drink some camomile before you go to bed,' she suggested.

'And the stiff joints? What can I do for those?' I asked.

'Yoga's very good at easing stiff joints and aching muscles. You'll find yourself loosening up again very quickly,' Dr Jones reassured me, before telling me to make another appointment to see her the same time next month, around the 18th February.

My heart leapt as she said the date. The eighteenth of February. That would make it a year since I was diagnosed. A whole year.

On my way home, I bought myself a Yoga video and an exercise mat, in order to do more yoga by doing it at home. I got up an extra half hour earlier and religiously did my exercises. It was a shock on the first day, as my body had seized up so much that I could barely lean forward, backward or sideways but as the months passed, I surpassed all personal expectations. I found myself leaning sideways as far as the girls on the video, and could touch my toes for the first time in years. And I started toning up a tiny bit. Not much, as I really needed to diet to lose weight as well as exercise.

That evening we went to The Wharf in Teddington with Colin's brothers and some friends – to celebrate Colin's 40th birthday.

February 2001

But despite my healthy regime, I was feeling really low. My mind kept preying on the events of the previous year. Each day, I drew a parallel with what I had been doing this time last year. On 9th February 2000 I was supposed to be flying to Thailand for a client meeting, which had been cancelled at the eleventh hour on the Tuesday night, which resulted in my keeping my appointment to see Dr Boxer. On Friday 11th I'd had a meeting with another client up near Aylesbury, and we had chatted about how overworked we were and the long hours we were putting in. The little landmarks that dated the calendar up to the day that changed my life so radically on 18 February 2000.

When I went to see Dr Jones on the 20th February, I was pleased to report that my joints were easing up. We chatted for a while, but I was feeling extraordinarily tense and unable to communicate with her – despite the fact that usually I found her very easy to talk to. I was just about to take my leave when Dr Jones suddenly said, 'Are you alright?'

Fatal. There are moments when that question is the worst possible question. I cracked, and burst into tears. I had no idea why. I thought I'd felt fine when I arrived at the appointment.

'If it helps, I know why you're feeling so miserable,' Dr Jones said kindly, pushing a box of tissues towards me.

'You do?' I looked at her, unsurprised, as she seemed to have all the answers.

'Most of the women I treat get miserable at the first anniversary.'

'The first anniversary?'

'Since you were diagnosed,' she looked at my notes. 'It was a year ago this week.'

'Oh I see. In fact, it *has* been playing on my mind. I've been reliving this time last year, the moment of diagnosis – looking at the detail, examining every memory I can recall,' I admitted. 'God only knows, I have enough wakeful hours in the night to ponder over it all.'

'Yes – and we're messing around with your hormones in a fairly major way. It's not really surprising that you'll feel emotional. Just make sure that you take it easy. I know you're back at work full time now, but don't overdo it. I mean it most seriously. You have to give your body *and* your mind time to repair – so don't start rushing back into things. And if you need someone to talk to, we have counsellors here that you can come and see.'

But already I was feeling mollified, just by knowing that my emotional state was probably grounded in hormone activity, as well as being a perfectly normal part of the process of getting past the first year. At last I could really put last year behind me, and look to the second year – a year of getting better.

> *Lesson learned:*
> **Focus on putting the whole experience behind you.**
> **Move on.**

Further reading "Life after cancer"
on the website www.careerkidsandbreastcancer.com

EPILOGUE

Five years later, I ask myself, was there a meaning in all of this? Has good come out of it, as so many people like to believe? I was certainly very overwhelmed in the months that immediately followed the completion of my treatment. So much had happened, yet I was trying to slot back into the life that I'd had before IT all happened. I couldn't think straight, and certainly was unable to put the whole experience into any form of perspective. So I decided to diarise the experience and put the completed document on a shelf for another time – for a time when I wanted to review that unexpected and shocking year in order to make some kind of sense of it all, to see what I had learnt, what the experience taught me and if there were any silver linings to that very dark cloud.

Hindsight often provides much clearer answers, so I left this question hanging for two years before I even attempted to define an answer. I have come up with answers each and every year over the last five years. Now, it is five full years since I was diagnosed with breast cancer. I am no longer being treated for cancer, and the most important knowledge that I have now is to LEAVE IT ALL BEHIND ME. So before I do, I want to just do "closure" on all my thoughts.

Putting it behind me!

The fact is, it has taken me all of five years to put this event behind me. After the first anniversary, I thought that was the beginning of the 'putting it behind me' phase but in fact that first year returning to work proved to be more of an emotional roller-coaster than the year of receiving treatment. I struggled to put the pieces of my life back to where they had been before the 18th February 2000, and stubbornly refused to accept that I had to create a new normality for myself. I was different. Cancer changes your views… I was more intractable as to how hard I would work, how many hours, how readily I would absorb other people's problems and laziness towards their work. Cancer changes other people's view of you... they tiptoe on eggshells, they remind you constantly (in a well-meaning way, I hasten to add). I was angry but had no-one to be angry at.

I fretted as to whether the cancer was coming back, and struggled to find a way to fit back into my old life whilst accommodating so many new influences and beliefs. How to work without overworking? How to do everything I wanted to do without filling up every second? How to learn to relax and switch off? How to learn to say No to extra demands on my time and energy?

Re-evaluating your life

People always say that you go through such a radical review and evaluation of your life when something like 'getting cancer' happens to you. And they talk about it in terms of making huge lifestyle changes, throwing up the expensive London house and top flight job to live a quiet life in the country growing vegetables; finding a more holistic lifestyle and shunning the commerciality of town life.

And that is what some people do. I didn't. My children were happy at their school. I was happy with my environment, lifestyle and local friends. My husband was happy with his job and his journey to work.

It was clear that something had to change, as something had gone horribly wrong but would I want to live remotely? I've lived in a village throughout my teenage years, and certainly there were benefits and it held its own charm. But all in all, I think country life would frustrate me – the fact that you can't just get a take-away food delivery day or night, or that you're endlessly in the car, or the post or milk is delivered late because the delivery van got stuck in a pothole down Mrs Robinson's driveway, or whatever. I think I've lived in the city, or suburbs, too long to now sacrifice all the conveniences that it brings. The children's school is one minute walk away, my office is fifteen minutes walk away, the shops are seven minutes walk and one of the biggest parks in London is eight minutes walk in the other direction.

I know this is detail, but convenience is good; I like convenience. And I certainly don't want to make change for changes sake. If I'm going to make any changes, I want them to be meaningful. I would happily move to the country in order to live in a large house with large garden, *if* my husband and I could reliably earn good incomes there. But I don't think I need to move to the country in order to learn how to manage stress and get a balance in my life – indeed, it would probably complicate our lives.

For me, a change of environment was the solution. I had to change something more fundamental within myself. I had lost a sense of perspective somewhere along the line, as my life was just about work, work, work. I woke up in the morning thinking about what I had to do that day, spent all day trying to achieve it whilst having thousands more tasks put in front of me, questions asked of me and challenges set in my path like an obstacle course. I was running around piling through chores each day, to have the next lot facing me like a new rack of ten pin bowls the next morning. I rampaged through them all, only to come home sometime between six thirty and seven, read a book at high speed to the children that was so summarised it probably no longer made sense, before staring at the television all evening.

I took on too much. I became superwoman, sorting out everyone else's problems. I filled in the gaps that other people couldn't, or just wouldn't, fill. I did their jobs for them. I did stuff that was unnecessary. I had lost the art of differentiating about what was worth doing and what was not worth doing. I set such a workload up in front of me that all I could do was run at it like a greyhound after the rabbit, blindly and with no real purpose.

And who benefited? A bunch of shareholders. Nobody I know.

And who lost out? Me. My husband. My children. This is not a way to make the family unit happy, and in my case this lifestyle also seriously undermined my health.

Lowering expectations

We live in a society of extremely high expectations – there's always more to have, to own, to upgrade to; not having these things leaves you feeling that you haven't achieved enough yet, or maybe even achieved anything at all. Success is relative to expectation. But at what price? When the most valuable thing you have is your life, why then beat the life out of yourself. You can't enjoy your life whilst slogging your guts out. I certainly was not spending enough time with my husband and children, and the time I did spend with them was often rushed, under scrutiny of a clock. Conversations were conducted at top speed, I didn't have time to play games with the children and I half-listened to Colin's account of his day whilst I mentally addressed the many questions running round my brain.

I wanted so much. I expected so much. And I had to lower my expectations in order to stop pushing myself so hard. It is fine to push yourself hard in bursts, but nobody can maintain such high standards on an ongoing basis. I have now learned to work at an even pace the majority of the time, with bursts of high activity to meet certain goals and objectives. It's a healthier way to approach work.

Returning to work was very difficult at first. My enforced time off work basically got in the way of my career plans, and it took me three full years to catch up to where I had been before. I tried to fit back in as though nothing had happened, whilst at the same time I was struggling to believe that I even had a future in front of me. I was no longer sure of what I was capable of, or what was being expected of me. I recommend that if you are returning to work, you get yourself a clear job description with clear expectations and targets to ensure both parties feel that a good job is being done. This reduces the stress caused by worrying whether you are fulfilling your role and management expectations of you. Again – expectations.

Precious precious time

Time is a commodity that you can't buy, yet you can sell it. Understand your value. Understand how much time you are prepared to sell and at what price. Then sell that. No more and no less. Then enjoy the time you set aside for yourself and your loved ones. That is the important thing. If you sell 7 hours of your time, then work for an extra 4 hours for free then you are a mug. The only person losing out is yourself. The only person benefiting are the people who share in profit-related bonuses – or the shareholders.

It is very difficult to be strict with your time. Everyone around you is busy working overtime. Directors expect it. Even the Government says that it is not going to enforce rigid working hours as they believe this 'loose' timekeeping in favour of businesses is what gives us such a lively economy.

However, after experiencing illnesses such as cancer, you HAVE to proceed cautiously. Not only is a state of cancer indicative of a low-functioning immune system, but also the chemotherapy drugs further suppress your immune system. It is all too easy to get sucked back into old behaviours and end up overdoing it. Despite all my good intentions, I have occasionally overdone it and become unwell as a result – shingles, migraines etc. But having had cancer FORCES me to change my ways as the price is too high a price to pay to ignore all the early warning systems. The change within me happens at a very fundamental level.

I now work four days a week with two afternoons off. This is enough to enable me to undertake a committed role at work, whilst giving me two afternoons with my children, being at the school gate, chatting to other mum's and teachers and generally being a part of my children's life. Children need help with forming friendships, and an active interest in their school life. They love seeing me at the school gate, and seeing my face in their world.

All I ever needed to do was to find the balance between work and home life, keeping the scales even rather than trying to do both 100% of the time and burning out.

Talking of time…

British society is in a bit of a mess right now. We have some major social issues which I believe stem from both parents working which leaves no time for children – let alone each other, house maintenance and domestic paperwork. These things don't go away but fester until they blow up in your face, which is happening in so many households today. Children can't bring themselves up. They need guidance and mentoring. They need time to be heard. They need to be understood and talked to. But society doesn't afford anyone time anymore. When are parents going to stop being so unrealistic to think that they can both work full time, flat out and raise socially-responsible children? When is society going to stop expecting them to work flat out?

Have faith, little one

The last two years have been tough in terms of retrieving the faith that I am well and that I have a life to live. For a long time I lived in a fear that some nasty little insidious cancer was growing silently inside me, but the misery this paranoia inflicted on me made it difficult to enjoy the life I had. I struggled to achieve a balance of work and home, trying to fit back into the many roles I filled before I got ill whilst worrying myself sick that I was overdoing it and going to make myself ill again.

I still struggle with this, and no doubt there will always be a little part of me that will be suspicious of certain 'signals'.

Analysing the treatments

Chemotherapy

I've said so much in the book, but suffice it to say that it really was not as bad as I was led to expect. But everyone's experience is different just as everyone's cancer is different – and maybe I was lucky in that respect.

Some people have asked me if I would use the ice-cap if I had to go through it all again. For a long time I said I wouldn't, but the years have changed my opinion and re-reading this diary also affects my view on this. It was another burden at a time of huge burden, but equally I didn't have to wear a wig from April through to November. My hair didn't look great, but there was hair. I would wear the ice-cap again.

Radiotherapy

This was a non-event in terms of how difficult the treatment was but I am the first to acknowledge that I was getting my treatment on private health. I had none of the hanging around which defines the national health service. I turned up each day at a given time, never waited more than five minutes, had the treatment and left. I suspect that my view of the actual process would be very different on the national health.

However, in defence of the national health, they put cancer treatment high on the agenda and apparently my initial surgery would have taken place within 24 hours of the private health date for surgery. Chemotherapy would have been the same type and the same dates. Ditto with radiotherapy. Dr Jones also reassured me that

Hormone treatments

The Zolodex has been more challenging, although fortunately the initial severe reaction eased off over the first six to eight months, and the injections themselves were made more bearable by having local anaesthetic injections rather than just an ineffectual cream. I have found that the effects of the Zolodex are more severe when I eat sugary foods, high carbohydrates and caffeine. So much so that I have lost all the extra weight I put on during the treatment and am now back at my initial weight before this upheaval began. I came off the Zolodex four months ago now. It's funny how the whole programme of treatment seemed to stretch before me at one point, and suddenly I am three years down the line and it is becoming a memory, rather than the present.

Telling the children

Do you tell them? Do you not? Cancer is a family issue. It impacts on everyone, and not even a young child can fail to sense the stress and upset. So do you tell them?

Grace was five and Eliot had just turned four in February 2000. I judged not to tell them explicitly as CANCER is a big and scary word. They were too young to understand that there were many different forms of cancer, different treatments and life expectancies. I haven't laboured my impression of Grace's fear (running downstairs at 6am to find me working on the computer, thinking I was dead) and Eliot's upset at school which the school chose to shield me from until a year later. They knew something was badly wrong at home. So do I think I should have been explicit?

No. I was right to eek information out slowly… in my view.

In April 2004, Grace finally asked me "Was it breast cancer you had?" I said yes, and explained it in full. I ask her, should I have told her when she was younger and she said "No. It would have really scared me. I knew you were ill, but not that ill."

We live in a world where we feel obliged to share adult concepts and knowledge with younger and younger children. But they are too immature to deal with it. Let them have a childhood, I say.

Diet & Nutrition

And what of all my investigations into diets and holistic living? Still all valid and interesting but you have to draw the line at some point and just live your life. I became as obsessed by diet and nutrition as I had always been about work. I think I need to learn to take a calmer, less obsessed view of life!

I certainly am considerably more informed about food than I ever was, and attempt to buy organic fruit, vegetables, dairy and meat whenever possible. My diet is so, so, so much healthier than it was before I ever got cancer, and hopefully this will rub off onto the children. It was difficult trying to learn how to embrace healthy living and eating into my whole approach, but now I have learned a new way of cooking and living, it is easy. It was merely the process of change that was difficult. And I remain convinced that this healthy approach works like the Tamoxifen, a small and consistent factor that works towards keeping my body free from cancer.

But whilst I try to buy organic food, I accept that I live in the world that I live, at a certain point in history where intensive farming with chemicals and meddling with the genetics of the food chain is rife. To avoid this touching your life, you would have to live in a very remote place and be totally self-sufficient.

I don't support governments who condone these farming practices, and I vote with my purse by buying organic, non-genetically modified food despite the premium prices. I fear for future generations of children, as I am sure tampering with the food chain will have a resounding impact. One just has to look at the spectrum of allergies and behavioural changes in children, and the increase in cancer (particularly hormone-related cancers) to know that there is an impact. But how much can one change one's life to avoid it. Different generations face a different set of challenges. Our generation faces threat from terrorism and war, AIDS and cancer… and don't even get me started on the drug-induced teenage rampage!

Intensive farming & Toxins

Whilst it is obvious there are dangers in ingesting all these chemicals, toxins, antibiotics and hormones, I think there are many real (and frequently overlooked) dangers present just in the amount of sugar we consume. Sugar problems exist all over the place – hyperactive children, increase in diabetes, increase in cancer etc. Ultimately the main change in my diet is to cut down on sugar and high fat carbohydrates – drastically. Chocolates, sweets, biscuits, pastries etc are treats to be consumed on special occasions. Ready meals just don't make it into my shopping basket, and refined products – white bread, pasta, rice etc - are eaten only on occasion.

However, there are times at work or in client meetings where only white bread and convenience canapés are served up. Do I eat it? Absolutely! Otherwise I'd end up going hungry!

It's just about moderation. I really faltered last summer, and by the end of August I was snacking between meals on sweets, cakes, crisps, biscuits etc, and I ballooned. A stone in one month! I felt bloated and puffy – it was awful. As soon as I stopped the high sugar, I 'deflated' again. I am now firmly of the belief that excess sugar *is* a toxin to my system. And by excess I mean regular, daily intake.

As a society, we live a pretty unhealthy life. We probably wouldn't be so ill if we all ate healthier - we could get the nation's NHS bill down to a fraction, just by having better nutritional information. When will we sit up and notice this, and start voting by shopping power? Stop buying all the ready meals and tinned/pre-packeted food that is filled with sugar. Go back to basics – buy vegetables that you have to chop, fruit you have to peel and meals you have to prepare and cook yourself.

Remember, the consumer has the ultimate power. We can buy it – or not! Only mugs buy the crap. Avoid all ready meals and high fat/high sugar foods. The volume of such rubbish will rapidly vanish from our shelves… or would you rather it stayed and tempted you?

Healthy living and eating

The main take out for me is that healthy living and eating is ultimately about prevention, rather than cure, and I continually work hard at trying to live a healthy lifestyle. I firmly believe the road to freedom and a longer future lies here. The shock for the world was when Kylie Minogue was diagnosed with breast cancer. Her perfectly formed figure, perfect skin, clear eyes and luscious hair – her whole brand message – shouts healthy living. Her diagnosis of breast cancer undermines everything we are led to believes. This rattled a lot of cages, including my own!

But will I turn to fags, copious alcohol, drugs, high fat, high sugar burgers, donuts and ready meals? Obviously not. I feel pretty good on a diet dominated by protein, fruit and veg irrespective of whether I look like Kylie or not. (And I don't).

The point that Mr Wintry was correctly making was that you can't cure yourself by diet – it's the medicine that cures – but the point he missed is that you can help PREVENT. This in itself is difficult to prove because if you prevent something happening, how do you know that it was ever going to happen? My answer – who cares to find out? Let's just eat and live healthily, then you know. You know that if you get ill, it wasn't because of a lack of effort on your part. You were given a body to live your life in, and you looked after it.

PS. On the subject of healthy living, in conjunction with the issue about anti-perspirants causing breast cancer, I have found a product called Crystal Fresh (available through most health shops). This is a deodorising stone that REALLY works. I have used it for two years now and never have body odour problems. I don't necessarily believe that anti-perspirants cause breast cancer, but feel that erring on the side of caution can only be a good thing.

My friend Sarah's story also rattles me. Sarah has done everything by the book to avoid the cancer coming back, then out of the blue I get an email advising me she has secondaries. How much can a person do? Honestly, not much more than Sarah.

Can a person then argue that they might as well eat the average American diet because if you're gonna get IT then you might as well enjoy yourself in the process? I just question whether a diet of Krispy Kreme donuts and life in a Fat-Chair is ultimately a life of enjoyment. I quite enjoy tennis on a Wednesday night and participating in the Mum's Run on Sports Day with my kids cheering me on. Do you want to spectate in life or participate? Sarah participated, and I am doing likewise.

Complementary therapies

And what about all the other complementary therapies? I think that there is validity in exploring all those avenues. I agree with Plato's 'mend the whole, not the parts' idea, and the fact that how can a body get well if a mind is unhappy, or not well. I think that the body and mind are inextricably linked, and that positive thinking will go a long way to aiding recuperation. I can only assume that that is the case for me. The 'conventional medical world' have blasted me with powerful chemicals and drugs and radiation, and continue to treat me with Tamoxifen which sits there tapping away at any cancerous cells that dare appear. In my turn, I have undertaken a wide range of complementary treatments.

It is difficult to measure the benefits of complementary therapies in the same way you can measure conventional treatments. Very few people survive on complementary therapies alone and those that do are the exception rather than the rule. BUT it may be more than we realise. Just because nobody funds long-term studies of the benefits of complementary treatments, doesn't mean the benefits aren't there. There's just more money pumped into researching success ratings with conventional medicines.

By complementary treatments I also include diet. To reiterate the sugar issue, it is my understanding that cancer thrives in a high sugar environment. By minimising my sugar intake, I am depriving any lurking cancer cells of their ability to thrive.

You experience a sense of empowerment when you work positively alongside the medical treatment. You feel optimistic, focused and motivated – in fact, I don't think I have ever been so focused on one challenge in my entire life. I shrugged off (with some difficulty) all other goals and objectives, and focused solely on getting my life back. By reading as voraciously as I did, and networking with all my friends and contacts, I gleaned so much information, all of which played its role in getting me through the treatment. Positive thinking plays a big role in cancer treatment - it energised me to change the unhealthy and stressful life I was living.

Counselling

Has the counselling been worth it? Following the Plato theory, I think that it is probably quite healthy to get an uninvolved third party view of your life at least once during your life, to show you new perspectives and allow you to look at your life from a different angle or viewpoint. Maybe it's helpful whenever you come to a crossroads in your life and you are trying to make life-changing decisions. Psychological analysis works when you look at the past to spot the patterns in your life that are caused by your behaviour / attitude / beliefs / personality, in order to learn, control and springboard forward. Personally, I believe that the moment you seek to dwell on the past, analysing too microscopically, does this type of counselling become destructive or negative.

- 0 -

The main thing is to put it all behind me. I finally feel that I have 'done cancer'. I have explored it from every conceivable angle, challenged it, questioned experts and read voraciously on research studies. Some of it will have rubbed off onto me, absorbing it into my everyday life subconsciously so that it is not an effort to put good habits into practice, whilst discarding elements that I believe are red herrings. I have survived over five years since that moment when I thought my days were numbered, and I am now impatient to just live my life normally again. The fact that I am no more reassured about my future than I was when this all started does not deflate me. Rather, it makes me realise that I must seek to achieve balances in my life. I will now finally reconsider what I expect to achieve in order to get the balance right.

So what good came out of the whole experience? For me, the changes are subtle on the outside, but fundamental on the inside. The experience enabled me to stop long enough to analyse the life I was living, the relationships I had with people close to me and the goals I had mentally set out ahead of me. In doing so, I found many silver linings, all of which existed before I was diagnosed, but I had neither stopped long enough to see them, nor nurtured them adequately in order to enjoy them as a part of my life.

The good is that the whole experience gave me time to put everything into perspective, to place values on aspects of my life, appreciate and emphasise the good and become more decisive in shaking off the bad, negative aspects of my life.

I debated whether or not to publish this diary. Would it be interesting to others? Or was it just the ramblings of my own experience, serving only to clarify my befuddled thoughts and therefore best consigned to the top shelf of my bookcase in manuscript format? However, my mind was made up when my friend Toddy called me asking for advice for a friend of hers who had been diagnosed with breast cancer. She was, like me, mid thirties with two young children yet the treatment she was offered was a fraction of the treatment I received.

This decided me. I firmly believe that through the surgery I received at Kingston Hospital and the oncology treatment from Dr Alison Jones' team at The Royal Free Hospital, I received the gold standard treatment available today. And this, must be every woman's right, to expect the same, if not better, treatment available. Treatments will change year on year, but should only ever build on the solid base of a gold standard. I just hope this book helps other people facing a diagnosis of breast cancer.

If you would like to share your experience with other people, go onto my website 'www.careerkidsandbreastcancer.com' and your experience may help someone else.

THANK YOU...

I want to take this opportunity to thank all the people that supported me during that year - and continue to support me either by direct medical care, or by their rationality in their advice and little demonstrations of care and support. It's always fatal to issue a list at this point, as somebody somewhere who did something that you really appreciated will be omitted. So I say to you that your kindness and/or advice was noted and appreciated with heartfelt thanks.

Heartfelt thanks to...

... Colin, my husband, an absolutely solid rock, whose rationality and support made the difference.

... Dr Boxer for referring me for screening, even when she didn't think there was anything to be alarmed about. It's conscientiousness like this that saves lives.

... Dr Alison Jones and her team - Teresa her assistant, Catherine Piggott the radiologist - for studying so hard at university in order to one day help me overcome a potentially fatal illness, for answering all the questions I asked, for treating me not just functionally but also emotionally.

... Mr Leach for his excellent surgery - the scars are barely visible.

... Mum, for constantly being there, dropping everything to help, saying the right things at the right time that hit the balance of sympathy and clear advice. Thanks for listening to the many rants and monologues at any & every time of the day and night, and for your particularly insightful advice whilst I tried to get my life back to normal.

...Grace and Eliot, for all your unconditional love and acceptance of the turmoil going on around you. You are both my little angels.

... James, Kate and Ian for the constant emails and phone calls that propped me up throughout that year (and since), the advice, the sympathy, the listening and just being there.

... Rita, who does so utterly much for me, Colin, the children and the running of the house; the children couldn't be better looked after, and I am so lucky to have so much support (all the other mothers at school constantly tell me how jealous they are). But also for your advice, endless listening to my analyses and knowing when (and when not to) be bossy.

... Granny and Grandad, for all your kind and wise words, cards and phone calls.

... Alice, for moving in next door, offering constant friendship and cups of coffee.

... Miranda, who rang regularly with recommendations on health & nutrition, emotional support and advice; for all your visits to see me, for saving Eliot from speeding a motorbike when my head was in the clouds, and also for mowing our lawn.

... Paul and Anne - for your advice, support and conversations, undoubtedly being a support to Colin; and also for a very, very relaxing and enjoyable day at the Sanctuary.

... Ray, for your support, visits & phone calls, enquiring after me regularly when you were going through your own difficult time; and for many Sunday lunches at TGI Fridays.

... to Toddy Crewdson, for her friendship over the years, your great sense of humour and a fun, relaxing weekend in Norfolk.

... to Peter and Anna Collins, for taking the time out to track down Dr Alison Jones, and for undoubtedly offering support to Colin in a way that I couldn't.

... Gary and Ashley Sandy, who again undoubtedly supported and helped Colin, as well as regular phone calls to check up on how I was; also for the photograph on the book jacket - I am flattered that some people think is me.

... to Viv and Richard Fowler, for phone calls, meals and trips to the hospital - and open-ended offers of help.

... to the mothers and teachers at St Luke's School who helped me and my children probably in more ways than I will ever know, as well as the help that I do know - picking children up, looking after them etc when I couldn't.

... to Lesley Bell, for that all-important first phone call and her very obvious desire to help other people.

... to Sarah Poulter, who has suffered likewise yet surprises the medical world with her success at fighting this illness of twice; and for listening to me prattle on!

... to everyone at work, to mention a few - Dave, Pete, Jo Saker, Gina, Kerry, Jason, Jenny, Alison, Kate, Jane, Clare, Hannah, Gail Turpin, Fiona McAnena, Nevine... the list is endless, for your flowers, cards, phone calls, lunches, advice and reassurance (not to mention being dumped with my workload when I disappeared so suddenly on the 18th February 2000).

... to Jo Dobson also for reiterating to me the importance of following a healthy diet at a time when I had become so utterly bored of not eating chocolate and cakes, and was slowly caving into temptation.

... to PPP for not making mountains out of molehills; the claim went through quickly and without fuss, and has done so since then.

... to CGNU for settling my critical illness insurance policy claim quickly and without fuss, as well as to Terry Metcalfe for selling me the insurance policy.

... Stan and Liz at the Firefly for providing such a lovely, secluded environment, great cocktails in a fun bar

... and everyone else who sent me cards and flowers, who rang me and/or Colin to offer works of sympathy & advice, took me out for lunch etc: Richard and Linda Jackson, Chloe and Polly Fowler, Alexis and Catherine Turner, Anne Ure, Kate and Clare Millington, my godmother Anne Corden who was suffering from cancer at the same time, and is still keeping well.

WHO DOES WHAT

Links on my website: www.careerkidsandbreastcancer.com

Breast Cancer Care: a nationwide charitable body that was founded to bring information and help to women with breast cancer. It offers emotional support counselling, answering questions and putting you in touch with one of 400 trained volunteers. There is a telephone support line for women with secondary breast cancer and a helpline for partners, as well as extensive free literature including a great leaflet on exercises to do following breast surgery to aid recovery and prevent the muscles seizing up. Helpline 0808 800 6000; Donation line 020 7384 4620

The Lavender Trust (in association with Breast Cancer Care) specialises in information for younger women with breast cancer; Helpline (as Breast cancer care); Donation line 020 7384 4617

Bristol Cancer Help Centre specialises in bringing complementary therapies to cancer patients, including self-help techniques and nutrition education, in order to aid self-healing; Helpline 0117 980 9505; Donation line 0117 980 9513

Cancer Bacup offers a comprehensive information service about cancer to patients and their families. Specialist nurses can answer questions on all types of cancer, they have an extensive list of publications and 2,000 pages of information on their website; Helpline 0808 800 1234; Donation line 020 7696 9003

The Haven Trust is a drop-in centre offering counselling, complementary therapies, advice and information, an extensive library, talks and meditative exercises such as yoga and Qi Gong; Helpline 020 7384 0099; Donation line 020 7384 0000

Macmillan Cancer Relief was founded to help prevent and relieve the suffering of patients. Macmillan nurses care for patients at home and in hospital offering everything from information, practical nursing help and advice on treatment to pain control for very ill patients;   Helpline 0845 6016161; Donation line 0845 60161616

Tenovus: set up to provide finance for hospital equipment, funds research into prevention and treatment of cancer, and offers counselling services from a team of nurses and social workers; Helpline 0808 800 1010; Donation line 02920 621433

CancerNet: a website gateway to the most recent and accurate cancer information from the National Cancer Institute (NCI) in America:

The Researchers
Breakthrough Breast Cancer: launched in 1991 to raise finance for breast cancer research. So far it has raised £15million, which funds campaigns to keep breast cancer a topline Government health priority; Telephone 020 7405 5111; Donation line 020 7405 5111

Cancer Research UK: the first cancer research institute founded in 1902, and now carries out one third of all cancer research in the UK. It works on anticancer vaccines, immunotherapy, and the development of smart drugs which targets cancer cells; Telephone: tel. 020 7242 0200

Cancer Research UK Events & Fundraising - 08701 60 20 40

Breast Cancer Campaign funds research into breast cancer and has so far received 25 research grants for scientific projects including younger women risk analysis, invasive breast cancer and resistance to Taxol treatments; Telephone 020 7749 3700; Donation line 020 7749 3700